Self-Assessment in
Paediatrics

Edited by

Tom Lissauer MB BChir FRCPCH
Honorary Consultant Paediatrician, Imperial College Healthcare Trust, London, UK
Centre for International Child Health, Imperial College London UK

Will Carroll BM BCh MD FRCPCH
Consultant in Paediatric Respiratory Medicine,
University Hospital of the North Midlands, Stoke-on-Trent, UK

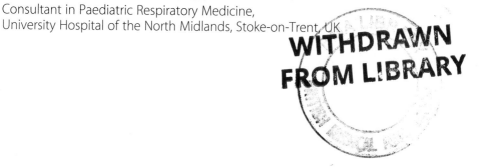

ELSEVIER

ELSEVIER

Notices

ISBN: 978-0-7020-7292-5
978-0-7020-7293-2

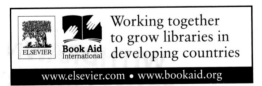

Working together
to grow libraries in
developing countries

www.elsevier.com • www.bookaid.org

Printed in Europe
Last digit is the print number: 9   8   7   6   5   4   3   2   1

Content Strategist: Pauline Graham
Content Development Specialist: Fiona Conn
Project Manager: Anne Collett
Design: Miles Hitchen
Illustration Manager: Amy Faith Heyden
Illustrator: Vicky Heim and TNQ
Marketing Manager: Deborah Watkins

Contents

Preface

The aim of this book is to consolidate knowledge of paediatrics and aid revision for examinations. The questions accompany the *Illustrated Textbook of Paediatrics* (5th edition), which contains all the core information on which the questions are based. It is primarily designed for medical students, however, it should also be a helpful revision aid for candidates preparing for postgraduate paediatric examinations, such as the Foundation of Practice component of the Membership of the Royal College of Paediatrics and Child Health examination or the Diploma of Child Health. Answers are provided for all questions, with additional comments or explanation to assist with understanding and learning about the topic and not just checking if the answer is right or wrong.

We have used two question formats, the Single Best Answer and Extended Matching Question. This reflects a change in examination assessment, with less use of multiple true-false questions. We have also included some illustrations to assess recognition of clinical conditions or interpretation of investigations.

While some of the questions test knowledge, we have also tried to assess understanding and decision-making. We have concentrated on the most important topics in paediatrics and have avoided rare problems unless an important message is conveyed. Our experience and feedback from many undergraduate medical schools in the UK, Europe, the Middle East, Hong Kong, Malaysia, Singapore, Australia and New Zealand, and Africa is that the *Illustrated Textbook of Paediatrics* and these self-assessment questions cover the range and depth of topics of the paediatric curriculum.

We very much hope that you will find the questions helpful in your revision and welcome feedback. And good luck in your examinations!

Tom Lissauer and Will Carroll

Acknowledgements

We have drawn extensively on questions and answers written for 'Illustrated Self Assessment in Paediatrics' by Tom Lissauer, Graham Roberts, Caroline Foster and Michael Coren (Elsevier, 2001) and modified by Peter Cartledge, Caroline Body, Elizabeth Waddington and Claire Wensley (https://studentconsult.inkling.com.2012) and wish to acknowledge and thank them for their contribution.

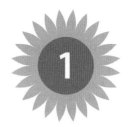

The child in society

1.1

Poverty is associated with the greatest increased risk of which one of the following conditions during childhood in the UK?

Select one answer only

A. Asthma
B. Cystic fibrosis
C. Developmental dysplasia of the hip
D. Febrile seizures
E. Pneumonia

1.2

Which of the following statements best describes the negative effects of poverty on child development?

Select one answer only

A. Especially harmful from the ages of birth to 5 years
B. More likely in the first child
C. Most pronounced in children from minority ethnic groups
D. Rare in developed countries like the UK
E. Temporary and resolve if familial poverty is addressed

1.3

In which age range is childhood mortality greatest?

Select one answer only

A. <1 year
B. 1–5 years
C. 5–9 years
D. 10–14 years
E. 15–19 years

Answers: Single Best Answer

1.1
A. Asthma ✓
Correct. Asthma shows a marked relationship with poverty as does low birthweight, injuries, hospital admissions, behavioural problems, special educational needs and child abuse. The relationship between poverty and other health problems is less clear cut.

B. Cystic fibrosis
A purely genetic condition; varies with ethnicity but not poverty.

C. Developmental dysplasia of the hip
This is a congenital disorder of unknown aetiology. It is more common in girls, if there is a family history, and breech presentation during pregnancy.

D. Febrile seizures
There is no socioeconomic influence.

E. Pneumonia
Within the UK and the developed world, the association is lost. However, in developing countries the risk is higher in those with malnutrition.

1.2
A. Especially harmful from the ages of birth to 5 years ✓
Correct. Research indicates that being poor at both 9 months and 3 years of age is associated with increased likelihood of poor behavioural, learning and health outcomes at age 5 years.

By the age of 4 years, a development gap of more than 1.5 years can be seen between the most disadvantaged and the most advantaged children. Babies whose development has fallen behind the norm during the first year of life are much more likely to fall even further behind in subsequent years rather than catch up with those who have had a better start.

B. More likely in the first child
Birth order has little effect. Singletons may have some protection as they do not have to compete for parental attention.

C. Most pronounced in children from minority ethnic groups
Whilst poverty is more common in minority ethnic groups the effects are similar across all groups.

D. Rare in developed countries like the UK
The UK has a higher proportion of children living in relative poverty than many countries in the European Union.

E. Temporary and resolve if familial poverty is addressed
We remain a hostage to our early life experiences. Paediatricians should act as advocates for the alleviation of childhood poverty.

1.3
A. <1 year ✓
Correct. Over half of deaths in childhood occur in infancy. Major causes are immaturity and congenital abnormalities.

History and examination

Questions: Single Best Answer

2.1
Ritha, aged 2 months, is admitted to hospital with a 2-day history of mild coryza and tachypnoea without significant intercostal recession. She has been feeding poorly for the last 3 weeks.

Which clinical feature most supports her having congenital heart disease rather than respiratory disease?

Select one answer only.

A. Sibling with congenital heart disease
B. Poor feeding
C. Generalized wheeze on auscultation
D. Hepatomegaly
E. Ejection systolic murmur, grade II/VI, at the left sternal edge

2.2
Nazma, aged 4 years, presents with a 1-week history of episodic central abdominal pain. She is of Indian ethnicity, but the family live in Kenya and are visiting relatives in the UK. She is otherwise well. Her relative's general practitioner thinks she may be slightly pale and that her spleen is enlarged, as it is 3 cm below the costal margin. There are no other abnormalities on examination.

Which of the following is the most likely cause for her enlarged spleen?

Select one answer only.

A. Acute lymphoblastic leukaemia
B. Malaria
C. Hookworm infestation
D. Wilms tumour
E. Sickle cell disease

2.3
Katie, an 18-month-old girl, is reviewed in the paediatric clinic. She is unsteady on her feet but has normal vision and gaze. She walks with a limp and tends to fall to her left side. Her limb tone and reflexes are as shown in Fig. 2.1.

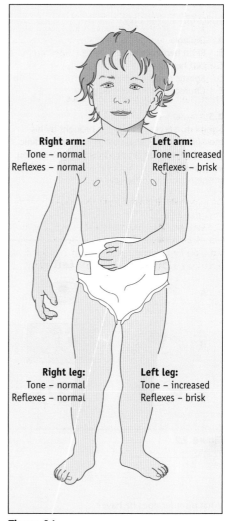

Right arm:
Tone – normal
Reflexes – normal

Left arm:
Tone – increased
Reflexes – brisk

Right leg:
Tone – normal
Reflexes – normal

Left leg:
Tone – increased
Reflexes – brisk

Figure 2.1

Which is the site of her neurological lesion?

Select one answer only.

A. Upper motor neurone lesion
B. Lower motor neurone lesion
C. Cerebellar lesion
D. Basal ganglia lesion
E. Neuromuscular junction

2.4
Katie's clinical problem and examination are described in Question 2.3.

Which of the following best describes the pattern of neurological signs?

Select one answer only.

A. Diplegia
B. Right hemiplegia
C. Left hemiplegia
D. Spastic quadriplegia
E. Choreoathetoid cerebral palsy

2.5
Jeremiah, a 6-year-old boy, is brought by his mother to the ophthalmology outpatient clinic. She is worried about her son's 'funny eyes'. You examine him using the cover test, and you find the signs shown in Fig. 2.2.

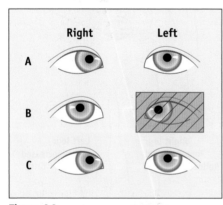

Figure 2.2

What disorder does he have?

Select one answer only.

A. Right convergent squint
B. Right divergent squint
C. Alternating convergent squint
D. Left convergent squint
E. Left divergent squint

2.6
William, a 9-year-old boy, presents to the rapid access paediatric clinic with a fractured tibia following a fall from a wall. He is otherwise well but has a history of shortness of breath and wheeze when running. His mother denies that he has ever needed treatment for his wheeze. He is not unwell currently.

What clinical sign is best shown in Fig. 2.3?

Select one answer only.

A. Barrel chest
B. Pectus excavatum
C. Pectus carinatum
D. Harrison sulcus
E. Sternal recession

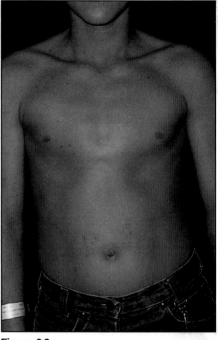

Figure 2.3

2.7
Ishmael, a 15-year-old boy from Pakistan, is seen in the outpatient department. He has a long history of chest infections needing recurrent courses of antibiotics. He has a productive cough. He opens his bowels once a day. On examination, he has a normal temperature, his skin and mucous membranes are pink and his heart sounds are normal. His hands look unusual (Fig. 2.4). On auscultation, there are some scattered crepitations at both bases. In view of his recurrent chest infections, you had ordered a sweat test, which is negative.

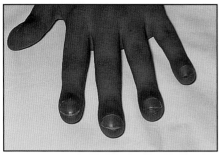

Figure 2.4

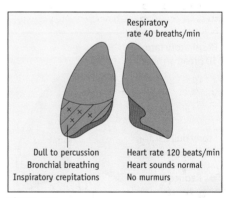

Figure 2.5

Which of the following is the most likely cause of the appearance of Ishmael's hands?

Select one answer only.

A. Cystic fibrosis
B. Infective endocarditis
C. Primary ciliary dyskinesia
D. Crohn's disease
E. Tetralogy of Fallot

Questions: Extended Matching

2.8
The following list (A–M) are causes of difficulty breathing in children. For each of the following clinical scenarios select the most likely diagnosis. Each answer may be used once, more than once or not at all.

A. Acute exacerbation of asthma
B. Bronchiolitis
C. Chronic asthma
D. Cystic fibrosis
E. Heart failure
F. Inhaled foreign body (left side)
G. Inhaled foreign body (right side)
H. Pleural effusion (left sided)
I. Pleural effusion (right sided)
J. Pneumonia (left sided)
K. Pneumonia (right sided)
L. Pneumothorax (left sided)
M. Pneumothorax (right sided)

2.8.1
Rob, a 9-month-old boy, presents with fever and difficulty breathing for the last 3 days. His breathing is now interfering with his feeding. He has not had any previous illnesses and his growth is normal.

Examination of his chest is shown in Fig. 2.5.

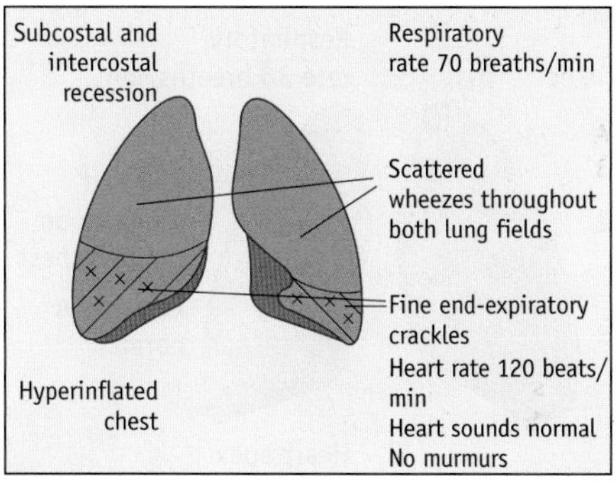

2.8.2
Hatem, a 3-year-old boy, presents with fever and difficulty breathing, getting worse for the last 3 days. Examination shows the clinical signs shown in Fig. 2.6.

Figure 2.6

2.8.3
Darren, a 3-year-old boy, was eating peanuts 2 days ago when his younger brother pushed him over. He coughed up the peanuts and was all right. Today, he has been coughing and becomes breathless as soon as he runs about. He is afebrile. Examination findings are shown in Fig. 2.7.

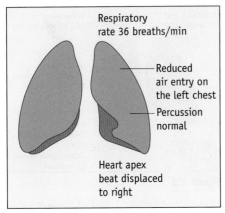

Respiratory
rate 36 breaths/min

Reduced
air entry on
the left chest

Percussion
normal

Heart apex
beat displaced
to right

Figure 2.7

2.8.4

Tony, a 4-year-old boy, is admitted with pneumonia. His chest X-ray shows consolidation at the right base. Despite antibiotic therapy, he remains febrile and unwell. Examination findings are shown in Fig. 2.8.

2.9

The following list (A–M) are causes of difficulty breathing in children. For the following clinical scenario select the most likely diagnosis.

A. Asthma
B. Bronchiolitis
C. Cystic fibrosis
D. Heart failure
E. Inhaled foreign body (left side)
F. Inhaled foreign body (right side)
G. Pleural effusion (left sided)
H. Pleural effusion (right sided)
I. Pneumonia (left sided)
J. Pneumonia (right sided)
K. Pneumothorax (left sided)
L. Pneumothorax (right sided)
M. Viral-induced wheezing

2.9.1

Jamalah, a 7-year-old girl, presents with difficulty breathing. She has had a cold for the last 2 days. This is the third time this has happened, each time when she had a cold. She has not had any other medical problems but her mother has noticed she 'coughs and whistles' when she goes out in the cold. On examination, she has an upper respiratory infection and the signs shown in Fig. 2.9.

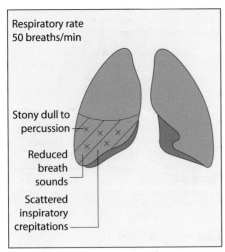

Respiratory rate
50 breaths/min

Stony dull to
percussion

Reduced
breath
sounds

Scattered
inspiratory
crepitations

Figure 2.8

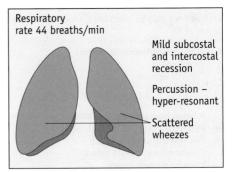

Respiratory
rate 44 breaths/min

Mild subcostal
and intercostal
recession

Percussion –
hyper-resonant

Scattered
wheezes

Figure 2.9

Answers: Single Best Answer

2.1

A. Sibling with congenital heart disease
A sibling with congenital heart disease slightly increases the risk for Ritha, but it is still very low.

B. Poor feeding
Poor feeding may be a clinical feature of either congenital heart or respiratory disease. The 3-week history may be related to her developing heart failure.

C. Generalized wheeze on auscultation
Generalized wheeze on auscultation may be a clinical feature of either congenital heart or respiratory disease.

D. Hepatomegaly ⊘
Correct. In infants, hepatomegaly is an important sign of heart failure, usually secondary to congenital heart disease. Heart failure can result from inadequate cardiac output (forwards failure) or failure to pump enough blood away from the system feeding it (backwards heart failure). In adults, left ventricular failure predominates, but in children either ventricle can fail.

E. Ejection systolic murmur, grade II/VI, at the left sternal edge
Ejection systolic murmur, grade II/VI, at the left sternal edge in isolation is most likely to be an innocent murmur.

2.2

A. Acute lymphoblastic leukaemia
Acute lymphoblastic leukaemia may cause splenomegaly, but other clinical manifestations would also be present.

B. Malaria ⊘
Correct. High prevalence in Kenya and may cause chronic anaemia and splenomegaly.

C. Hookworm infestation
Hookworm infestation is associated with anaemia but not splenomegaly.

D. Wilms tumour
Wilms tumour would cause enlarged kidney rather than spleen.

E. Sickle cell disease
Sickle cell disease may cause anaemia and splenomegaly, but prevalence is very low in Indian ethnicity, whereas malaria is common in Kenya.

2.3

A. Upper motor neurone lesion ⊘
Correct. The increased tone and reflexes of her left arm and leg are from an upper motor neurone lesion, most likely in the right side of her brain.

B. Lower motor neurone lesion
Tone and reflexes would be decreased.

C. Cerebellar lesion
Cerebellar signs would be found including nystagmus, past-pointing, and ataxia.

D. Basal ganglia lesion
There would be abnormal limb movements.

E. Neuromuscular junction
This is a lower motor neurone lesion, and signs would therefore include decreased tone and reflexes.

2.4

A. Diplegia
This affects all four limbs, the lower limbs more than the upper limbs.

B. Right hemiplegia
Right hemiplegia describes the abnormal clinical signs in the limbs, not the affected side of the brain. Katie's left limbs are affected, so she does not have a right hemiplegia.

C. Left hemiplegia ⊘
Correct. Katie has a left hemiplegia due to the increased tone and reflexes on her left arm and leg.

D. Spastic quadriplegia
Spastic quadriplegia is when all four limbs are affected, often severely.

E. Choreoathetoid cerebral palsy
There are abnormal movements of the limbs.

2.5

A. Right convergent squint ⊘
Correct. It is a convergent squint because the eye is facing inwards towards the midline. It affects the right eye when both eyes are uncovered. The uncovered left eye usually focuses on objects. But when the left eye is covered, the right eye takes up a normal position and focuses.

B. Right divergent squint
In a divergent squint, the eye deviates laterally away from the midline.

C. Alternating convergent squint
The left eye would remain convergent after uncovering.

D. Left convergent squint
The left eye is fixing until it is covered up, and therefore is not squinting.

E. Left divergent squint
The left eye is fixing until it is covered up, and therefore is not squinting.

2.6

A. Barrel chest
A barrel chest is hyperinflated with a large anterior–posterior measurement to look like a round barrel.

B. Pectus excavatum
This is when there is a hollow in the anterior chest wall.

C. Pectus carinatum
This is a defect of the anterior chest wall caused by bulging of the sternum (pigeon chest).

D. Harrison sulcus ⊘
Correct. Harrison sulcus is caused by chronic indrawing of the chest wall because of diaphragmatic tug from chronic respiratory disease. In this case he appears to have chronic under-treatment of asthma.

E. Sternal recession
Sternal recession is an acute sign of respiratory distress and is not consistent with the history given above.

2.7
A. Cystic fibrosis
This is effectively excluded by a negative sweat test.

B. Infective endocarditis
Ishmael has no fever and examination does not support this diagnosis.

C. Primary ciliary dyskinesia ⊘
Correct. This child has marked clubbing of the fingers due to bronchiectasis. Although cystic fibrosis is the commonest cause of clubbing due to respiratory disease, it may also be caused by other respiratory conditions including primary ciliary dyskinesia.

D. Crohn's disease
Ishmael has no gastrointestinal symptoms.

E. Tetralogy of Fallot
If Ishmael had tetralogy of Fallot, he would be cyanosed and have an abnormal cardiac examination.

Answers: Extended Matching

2.8.1
B. Bronchiolitis
The child's age, history, and clinical signs are characteristic of bronchiolitis. The signs are bilateral, which excludes unilateral lesions. Heart failure is unlikely as cardiac examination is normal and there is no hepatomegaly.

2.8.2
K. Pneumonia (right sided)
This child has 'classic' signs of a right-sided pneumonia. Stony dullness (rather than just dullness to percussion) would suggest fluid accumulation – a pleural effusion. Percussion is possible in most children.

2.8.3
F. Inhaled foreign body (left side)
In clinical practice, 50% of children with inhaled foreign body do not volunteer a history of inhalation. In this case, there is reduced air entry on the left side and heart apex beat displaced to the right, suggesting that the peanut has eventually ended up in the left bronchus with reduced air entry on inspiration and a ball-valve effect causing hyper-expansion distally causing the apex beat to be displaced to the right. It is most common for foreign bodies to initially descend down the straighter, wider right main bronchus and lodge here. However, inhaled nuts can 'move around' in the larger airways as coughing can dislodge them.

2.8.4
I. Pleural effusion (right sided)
The signs are of a right pleural effusion.

2.9.1
A. Asthma
Whilst not all that wheezes is asthma, this is a common diagnosis and the most likely in this scenario. In clinical practice, it is helpful to distinguish between viral-induced wheeze and asthma as the latter is steroid-responsive. Young children with asthma typically have interval symptoms (wheezing and cough when well), as described by Jamalah's mother, and most have atopy (eczema). Lung function tests are diagnostic and usually possible in children of 7 years.

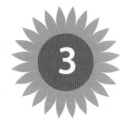

Normal child development, hearing and vision

Questions: Single Best Answer

3.1
Steven has just had his first birthday party. During his party he commando crawled with great speed, although he cannot walk. He managed to pick off all the Smarties (round chocolate sweets) from his birthday cake. He can say two words with meaning. After his birthday party, he impressed his guests by waving goodbye.

Which area of Steven's development is delayed?

Select one answer only.

A. Fine motor and vision
B. Gross motor
C. Social, emotional and behavioural development
D. Speech and hearing
E. None – his development is within normal limits

3.2
Gerald is a 16-month-old boy who has not yet said his first word and does not babble much. His mother believes he does not hear well because he does not startle when a door slams or show any response to his name. His development is otherwise normal.

Which test would be best to assess Gerald's hearing?

Select one answer only.

A. Auditory brainstem response audiometry
B. Distraction hearing test
C. Otoacoustic emission
D. Speech discrimination testing
E. Visual reinforcement audiometry

3.3
Evie is a 10-day-old infant and was born in London. Her health visitor reviews the family at home. She is feeding well and has a normal examination except that she has a squint. The health visitor tells her parents that she will keep this under review.

At what age does Evie need to be referred for further review if the squint is still present?

Select one answer only.

A. 2 weeks
B. 6 weeks
C. 12 weeks
D. 8 months
E. 12 months

3.4
Sophie is a well 8-week-old baby who was born at term. She has come for a routine developmental check.

Which of the following would you NOT expect her to be able to do?

Select one answer only.

A. Auditory brainstem response audiometry
B. Fix and follow a toy
C. Quieten to a loud noise
D. Raise her head when lying prone
E. Reach out and grasp an object

3.5
Joanna is an active toddler. She is just being potty trained and has had several days where she has remained dry. She enjoys pulling her clothes off to use the potty but cannot dress herself again. She enjoys playing by pretending to make her mother a cup of tea but does not play well with her older siblings, as she has not yet learnt how to take turns. She is very bossy and demands things by saying 'give me' or 'me drink'. She can build a tower of six blocks and enjoys running and climbing on furniture.

What developmental age is Joanna?

Select one answer only.

A. 12 months
B. 18 months
C. 24 months
D. 2.5 years
E. 3 years

3.6

Cordelia is a 4-month-old baby girl who is assessed by her general practitioner because of constant crying and poor feeding. She is fed by bottle on infant formula. Her mother tearfully complains that she is finding it very difficult to cope. She also has a 20-month-old son who has recently been referred to the speech and language therapist because of language delay. Charlotte's development, growth and physical examination are normal.

What is the likely cause of Cordelia's problems?

Select one answer only.

A. An inherited genetic condition
B. Cow's milk protein allergy
C. Down syndrome
D. Gastro-oesophageal reflux
E. Maternal postnatal depression/stress

Questions: Extended Matching

3.7

At what age would one expect children to achieve the milestones described in the scenarios (median age) described below? Each age can be used once, more than once, or not at all.

A. 6 weeks
B. 6 months
C. 8 months
D. 10 months
E. 12 months
F. 18 months
G. 2 years
H. 3 years
I. 4 years
J. 5 years

3.7.1
Rosette can build a three-cube tower and can point to her nose.

3.7.2
Peace has just taken her first steps!

3.7.3
Anthony has a friend at nursery, and they enjoy playing with toy cars together.

3.7.4
Herbert can transfer objects from one hand to the other whilst sitting without support and with a straight back.

3.7.5
Grace enjoys drawing. She has just learnt to copy drawing a square, and can build steps using blocks after being shown.

3.7.6
Rita's father is thrilled that she has just said her first word – says 'dada' to her father only.

3.7.7
Rinah can follow her mother's two-step commands, such as 'Go to the cupboard and fetch your red shoes'.

3.7.8
Blessing's mother is so pleased; her baby has just learnt to smile when she smiles at her!

3.7.9
Ivan can tie his shoe laces all by himself.

3.7.10
Lizzie has just started crawling.

3.8

At which of these ages is the following action (screening, examination, health promotion activity) usually first taken in the child health surveillance and promotion programme in the United Kingdom? Each answer can be used once, more than once, or not at all.

A. Newborn
B. 5–6 days
C. 12 days
D. 8 weeks
E. 3 months
F. 4 months
G. 8 months
H. 12 months
I. 2–3 years
J. 4–5 years (preschool)
K. 5 years (school entry)

3.8.1
First measles/mumps/rubella (MMR) immunization.

3.8.2
Biochemical screening test (Guthrie test).

3.8.3
Advice on reducing the risk of sudden infant death syndrome by 'back to sleep', avoiding overheating and avoiding parental smoking.

3.8.4
Hearing test using otoacoustic emission or auditory brainstem response audiometry.

3.8.5
An orthoptist assessment for visual impairment.

Answers: Single Best Answer

3.1

A. Fine motor and vision
Fine motor: he must be able to perform a pincer grip to be able to pick small chocolates off his birthday cake.

B. Gross motor
Gross motor: Steven commando crawls, so is expected to walk later than the median age of 12 months.

C. Social, emotional and behavioural development
Social: he can wave goodbye.

D. Speech and hearing
Speech: aged 1 year he is able to say two words with meaning.

E. None – his development is within normal limits ⊘
Correct. He has achieved normal milestones for a 12-month-old.

3.2

E. Visual reinforcement audiometry ⊘
Correct. This is the most reliable test for a child of Gerald's age. The test requires an assistant to play with the child and keep his attention. Behind a soundproof window, another assistant will play sounds through a loudspeaker at particular frequencies. When the child turns around to the noise, a glass-fronted box with a previously dark toy inside lights up as visual reinforcement to reward the child for turning around.

3.3

C. 12 weeks ⊘
Correct. Newborns may appear to squint when looking at nearby objects because their eyes over-converge. By 6 weeks of age, the eyes should move together when following an object, and by 12 weeks of age there should be no squint present.

3.4

A. Auditory brainstem response audiometry
Hearing in newborn children can be tested using this method.

B. Fix and follow a toy
A baby should be able to fix and follow either a face or a brightly coloured object by 6 weeks.

C. Quieten to a loud noise
Usually a baby can do this by 1 month of age. It is a useful question to ask parents if hearing is a concern.

D. Raise her head when lying prone
A 6 to 8 week old infant should be able to lift her head by 45°.

E. Reach out and grasp an object ⊘
Correct. An 8 week old infant will not be able to voluntarily reach out to grasp an object; she will only be able to grasp what is placed in her hand.

3.5

A. 12 months
The two-word sentences suggest that Joanna is more advanced than 1 year.

B. 18 months
A six-block tower would be advanced for 18 months.

C. 24 months ⊘
Correct. Joanna is dry by day, can undress, and has symbolic play. She is not yet playing interactively; she will learn this at about 3 years of age. She is constructing two word sentences. She constructs a tower of six blocks and can run. In assessing development, find the most advanced skill that cannot be performed.

D. 2.5 years
We would expect more in language development by 30 months.

E. 3 years
Joanna has imaginative play but is not yet playing interactively, as would be expected at this age.

3.6

A. An inherited genetic condition
Although more than one child is affected, besides genes they also share a home environment.

B. Cow's milk protein allergy
A common and important cause of distress in bottle-fed infants which should be suspected if there is eczema, family history of allergies and/or blood in the stool or faltering growth.

C. Down syndrome
The examination is normal.

D. Gastro-oesophageal reflux
A common diagnosis but there are hints of other issues. Why would this lead to speech delay in a sibling?

E. Maternal postnatal depression/stress ⊘
Correct. This may be detrimental to Cordelia's development, as infants are totally dependent on their main caregiver. Her older brother may have speech and language delay because he is not receiving enough stimulation to develop his own language skills or there may be an underlying problem causing his speech delay.

Answers: Extended Matching

3.7.1
F. 18 months
By 18 months can usually build a small tower of bricks and can point to several parts of the body.

3.7.2
E. 12 months
One year is the median age for children to walk (a few steps) and say two to three words. These are very important milestones.

3.7.3
H. 3 years
At 3 years, children develop interactive play and turn-taking. It may emerge slightly sooner in those who attend nursery or in those with siblings.

3.7.4
C. 8 months
Children transfer objects around 7 months of age. A rounded back requires control of T1 to T12, but a straight back requires T12 and L1 so develops later. A child will often 'sit' at 6 months but sit and be stable and with a straight back at 8 months.

3.7.5
I. 4 years
Asking a child to draw (copy) shapes is a good way of 'estimating' their age. They scribble first (age 2 years), then can copy a circle (by 3 years), and a square (by 4 years). A triangle (by 5 years) follows.

3.7.6
D. 10 months
Many children will make double-syllable sounds which are not specific to an object or person. In this case, the word 'dada' is specific for her father and so indicates 10 months of age.

3.7.7
H. 3 years
At about 2½ years of age, children can follow a two-step set of instructions. It is important to

make sure it is a true 'two-step' command. Children may fetch a toy (one-step command) if they know where it is.

3.7.8
A. 6 weeks
An important and remarkably constant milestone.

3.7.9
J. 5 years
You might remember being 'taught' this skill! It is acquired at a variable age but requires good fine motor skills and 'memorization' of the task. Most children can do this by the time they finish their first year of primary school education in the UK.

3.7.10
C. 8 months

3.8.1
H. 12 months
It is usually given at 12 months in the UK.

3.8.2
B. 5–6 days
Screens for congenital hypothyroidism, cystic fibrosis, haemoglobinopathies and a range of inborn errors of metabolism. Some of the inborn errors of metabolism cannot be detected until metabolites have accumulated. Therefore, the age at which the test is done is a compromise, as some infants may present before day 5 of life.

3.8.3
A. Newborn
This advice should also be given throughout pregnancy.

3.8.4
A. Newborn
Performed in the neonatal period. Undertaking this whilst still in hospital ensures that few children miss their screening.

3.8.5
J. 4–5 years (preschool)
This should be performed prior to starting school.

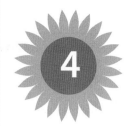

Developmental problems and the child with special needs

Questions: Single Best Answer

4.1

Jonathan is 4 years old and lives in a small village in southern England. He attends a paediatric outpatient clinic with his grandmother who is his legal guardian. She is concerned that he only seems to like to play with his toy train and insists on watching the same DVD every night before he goes to bed. He attends nursery where he plays with the toys but not with other children. His behaviour can be very difficult to manage at times. He does not say any words, whereas the grandmother's children were speaking in sentences at his age. On examination you notice he does not make eye contact with you and pushes his toy train back and forth on the floor. The rest of his examination is normal.

What is the most likely diagnosis?

Select one answer only.

A. Asperger syndrome
B. Attention deficit hyperactivity disorder
C. Autism spectrum disorder
D. Developmental coordination disorder (also known as dyspraxia)
E. Expressive language disorder

4.2

At what age does autism spectrum disorder usually become evident?

Select one answer only.

A. 0–12 months
B. 12–24 months
C. 2–4 years
D. 4–8 years
E. Above 8 years

4.3

At what age would you expect the clinical features of spastic bilateral cerebral palsy to become evident?

Select one answer only.

A. 0–12 months
B. 12–24 months
C. 2–4 years
D. 4–8 years
E. Above 8 years

4.4

Fortuna is an 8-month-old black African girl who was born at term. She is seen in the paediatric outpatient department. She can roll over. She does not crawl. She can say 'dada', but says it to everyone not just her father. She reaches out and grasps objects with her left hand but not with her right, and puts objects in her mouth. She smiles, but is not able to wave bye-bye.

Which aspect of her development is of most concern?

Select one answer only.

A. Does not wave bye-bye
B. Inability to crawl
C. Inability to use sounds discriminately to parents
D. Left-hand preference
E. None of the above

4.5

Gloria is a 19-month-old girl who presents to you in primary care. Her health visitor is concerned because she is still only babbling and says no distinct words. She is able to walk, scribbles with crayons and feeds herself with a spoon.

What is the most appropriate first action?

Select one answer only.

A. Hearing test
B. Assessment by a team specializing in autism spectrum disorders
C. Reassure the health visitor
D. Refer to an ear, nose and throat surgeon
E. Refer to a paediatrician for a full developmental assessment

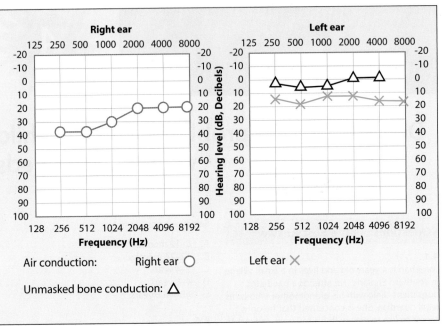

Figure 4.1

4.6

Andrew is a 5-year-old boy. His father feels his behaviour has deteriorated and he is worried he is not hearing him all the time. He has poor articulation of the few words that he can say. Andrew goes to the audiology department and has his hearing tested. His audiogram is shown in Fig. 4.1.

What type of hearing loss does he have?

Select one answer only.

A. Mild conductive hearing loss in the right ear
B. Mild sensorineural hearing loss in the right ear
C. Mixed hearing loss in the right ear
D. Moderate sensorineural hearing loss in the right ear
E. Severe conductive hearing loss in the right ear

4.7

Cruz is a 2-year-old boy. He has recently moved to the UK from Mexico. He attends the audiology department as he has marked problems with his language development. His audiogram is shown in Fig. 4.2.

What type of hearing loss does he have?

Select one answer only.

A. Mild conductive hearing loss in both ears
B. Mild sensorineural hearing loss in both ears
C. Mixed hearing loss in both ears
D. Severe conductive hearing loss in both ears
E. Severe sensorineural hearing loss in both ears

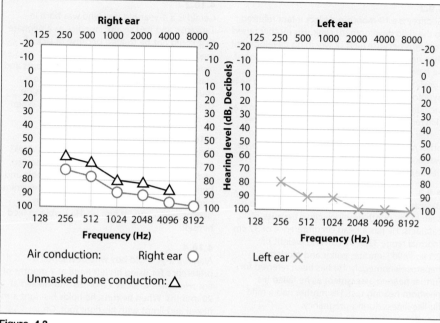

Right ear

Left ear

Hearing level (dB, Decibels)

Frequency (Hz)

Air conduction: Right ear ○ Left ear ✕

Unmasked bone conduction: △

Figure 4.2

4.8

Jenny is an 8-week-old girl who was born preterm at 35 weeks' gestation. She is seen by her general practitioner for her surveillance review. Her mother is concerned that she does not smile. Her gross motor development appears to be normal and she startles to loud noises. However, she will not follow a face or a colourful ball. The appearance of one of her eyes is shown in Fig. 4.3. The other eye has a similar appearance. She has no other medical problems.

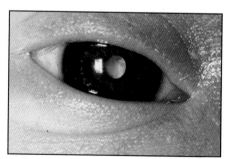

Figure 4.3

What is the likely underlying diagnosis?

Select one answer only.

A. Cataract
B. Conjunctivitis
C. Corneal trauma
D. Retinopathy of prematurity
E. Vitamin A deficiency

Questions: Extended Matching

4.9

Which of these investigations [A–J] would you choose to initially undertake to confirm the diagnosis of developmental delay in the children described in the following scenarios? Each investigation can be used once, more than once, or not at all.

A. Blood lactate
B. Chromosome karyotype
C. Congenital infection screen
D. Cranial ultrasound scan
E. Creatine kinase
F. CT or MRI scan of the brain
G. DNA fluorescent in situ hybridization (FISH) analysis
H. EEG
I. Maternal amino acids for raised phenylalanine
J. Thyroid function tests

4.9.1

Clarissa, a cheerful 20-month-old white British girl, is referred to the child development clinic by her health visitor because she is not yet walking. She was born at term with no complications. She learnt to sit without support at 10 months, and is able to crawl, although she drags her right leg behind her. Her mother says that she has always been left handed. Examination of the right arm and leg reveals reduced power but increased tone and reflexes.

4.9.2

Geoffrey is a 10-month-old black infant referred to the child development clinic. His mother raised concerns because he is slower in his development than her four other children. He can sit but only if he is propped up with cushions. He is not crawling or pulling to stand. On examination he is hypotonic, with some dysmorphic features, including upslanting palpebral fissures. There is a skin fold of the upper eyelid covering the inner corner of the eye and a flat occiput. He has no other medical problems except some vitiligo. He was born at term by normal vaginal delivery. He has been slow to feed.

4.9.3

Batar is a 1-week-old baby born at term who is seen in the ophthalmology clinic because of cataracts. He has a head circumference of 32 cm (normal range 32.5–37 cm) and weight of 2.3 kg, mild jaundice, pallor and moderate hepatosplenomegaly. He has been referred for further hearing assessment as he failed his newborn hearing test. His mother had a mild flu-like illness during pregnancy.

4.9.4

Dorcus, a 9-month-old infant, attends the clinic because of unusual movements. She has developed episodes of suddenly throwing her head and arms forward. These occur in repetitive bursts. She was able to sit and babble but has stopped doing so.

4.9.5

Darren is a 3-year-old boy who has difficulty climbing stairs. He always needs to hold on to the railings or to have a supporting hand. He walked unsupported at 14 months. His development is otherwise normal. On examination the power in his legs is reduced, he is somewhat hypotonic but his reflexes are normal.

4.10

Considering these types of cerebral palsy, choose the type of movement disorder to fit the following scenarios. Each type of cerebral palsy [A–E] can be used once, more than once, or not at all.

A. Dyskinetic
B. Ataxic
C. Spastic diplegia
D. Spastic hemiplegia
E. Spastic quadriplegia

4.10.1

Moses is a 5-year-old boy who failed to attain his developmental milestones from shortly after birth. Currently, he cannot roll or talk, but he can smile. His mother complains it is difficult to dress him as both his arms and legs are stiff. On examination, his left and right upper and lower limbs are stiff and hyperreflexic. He has a primitive grasp reflex in both hands.

4.10.2

Gerald is a 4-year-old boy who was born in Tanzania, and had severe jaundice as a neonate that could not be treated because of lack of medical services. He now has abnormal movements of all his limbs where he adopts and maintains unusual postures, and when he is startled by a loud noise, the arm on one side straightens and the opposite arm bends. When he is asleep he is hypotonic.

4.10.3

Hassan is 3 years old and was born at 26 weeks' gestation weighing 700 g. He sat at 10 months, and has just started to walk. He can scribble and build a tower of three blocks. When you examine him, he is walking on tiptoes, and his legs 'scissor' when you lift him up. He is able to feed himself.

4.10.4

Alan is a 3-year-old boy who developed a preference for using his left hand at 7 months of age. He learnt to sit at 9 months and walked at 20 months. When he runs, he holds his right arm flexed and limps with his right foot. On examination, his right upper and lower limbs are stiff, with increased reflexes.

4.10.5

Ronaldo is a 6-year-old boy. He attends the outpatient department as his teacher has had some concerns. He has recently started school and has been noted to be unsteady on his feet. He has to walk and run with his legs quite wide apart to stop himself from falling over. His teacher also reports that he finds it difficult to grip a pen and to write because of unsteadiness.

4.11

Which of the following health professionals (A–H) involved in the care of a disabled child would be of MOST help to the children described below?

A. Dietician
B. Occupational therapist
C. Paediatrician
D. Physiotherapist and occupational therapist
E. Psychologist
F. Social worker
G. Specialist health visitor
H. Speech and language therapist

4.11.1

Adrianna is a 4-year-old girl who has recently moved from Poland to the UK. She has severe learning difficulties and attends a special nursery. She has epilepsy, which is difficult to control, and is on two different anti-epileptic drugs. She continues to have seizures despite this medication. She does not have an underlying diagnosis.

4.11.2
Frankie is a 6-month-old infant.
She has always struggled to gain weight. On feeding she often had choking episodes which led to two episodes of pneumonia. She subsequently needed to have a nasogastric tube and gastrostomy so she could be fed. Her mother wants to start trying to feed her some solid food.

4.11.3
Sian is 2 years old. She is being followed up for growth faltering. All her investigations have come back normal but she is still not gaining adequate weight. She drinks a lot of dilute squash but her mother complains she will not eat any of the food she gives her.

4.11.4
Thomas is a 9-year-old boy who has suspected Asperger syndrome. He has problems interacting with his siblings and classmates. His academic performance at school is poor. He has a very strict daily routine and becomes very upset if this is broken. He sleeps poorly at night.

4.11.5
Bilal is a 5-year-old boy who has Duchenne muscular dystrophy. This presented with weakness and easy fatiguability when walking. He is in mainstream school and is finding it increasingly difficult to move around the classroom.

4.11.6
Gloria is a 22-month-old girl whose health visitor is concerned because she is still only babbling and says no distinct words. She is able to walk, scribbles with crayons, and feeds herself with a spoon.

4.11.7
Cathy is 15 years old and was in a road traffic accident. She spent a week in intensive care and needed an operation on her spine. She is currently not able to walk and has been shown how to use a wheelchair. Her parents are desperate to get her back home. They live in a town house where her bedroom is on the first floor, and therefore her father would need to carry her up the stairs.

4.11.8
Jake is a 20-month-old boy who burnt himself on a radiator whilst playing unsupervised. He attended the Accident and Emergency department where analgesia was given and dressings applied. He was seen by a paediatrician who performed a more detailed assessment for child abuse. There were no concerns and the child was discharged home to be seen later in the burns clinic.

Answers: Single Best Answer

4.1

A. Asperger syndrome
Children with Asperger syndrome have similar but less severe social impairments and near-normal language development.

B. Attention deficit hyperactivity disorder
Attention deficit hyperactivity disorder also presents with difficult behaviour but there is a triad of attention deficit, hyperactivity and impulsivity.

C. Autism spectrum disorder ⊘
Correct. Autism is a triad of impaired social interaction, speech and language disorder, and ritualistic and repetitive behaviour.

D. Developmental co-ordination disorder (also known as dyspraxia)
There are no signs of developmental co-ordination disorder reported.

E. Expressive language disorder
Here language alone is affected.

4.2

A. 0–12 months
Functional language has not developed yet.

B. 12–24 months
Concerns may emerge at this stage but problems are less obvious and overdiagnosis is a problem.

C. 2–4 years ⊘
Correct. Autism spectrum disorder usually presents at this age because this is when language and social skills rapidly develop.

D. 4–8 years
It is unusual to get to school before problems are noticed but this does occasionally happen.

E. Above 8 years
Minor symptoms and conditions such as Asperger syndrome may present later.

4.3

A. 0–12 months ⊘
Correct. Cerebral palsy most often presents during this time when acquisition of motor skills occurs most rapidly.

B. 12–24 months
As the child gets older, the increased tone becomes more evident.

C. 2–4 years
Most children with cerebral palsy have presented prior to this but very mild hemiplegia can be missed.

D. 4–8 years
Only very subtle problems will emerge in early school years.

E. Above 8 years
Unusual. Cerebral palsy is the result of a fixed insult usually in early life.

4.4

A. Does not wave bye-bye
Usually this skill develops at about 1 year.

B. Inability to crawl
Children begin to crawl at around 8 months but this would not be a worrying sign at this stage.

C. Inability to use sounds discriminately to parents
Functional expressive language begins at about 1 year.

D. Left-hand preference ⊘
Correct. Fortuna has developed a preference for using her left hand at 8 months. Development of hand preference before 1 year of age is abnormal.

E. None of the above
Although examination technique suggests that this is frequently the correct option, it is not in this case.

4.5

A. Hearing test ⊘
Correct. Speech delay can be due to hearing impairment and this should be assessed first prior to referring her to a specialist.

B. Assessment by a team specializing in autism spectrum disorders
Whilst autism is typified by expressive language difficulties this is only part of the problem.

C. Reassure the health visitor
The problem may resolve spontaneously but further action is required if no clear words have emerged by 18 months.

D. Refer to an ear, nose and throat surgeon
Grommets for conductive hearing loss might be the solution but it would be important to check hearing first.

E. Refer to a paediatrician for a full developmental assessment
The service would be impossibly busy if all children with speech delay at this age were immediately referred.

4.6

A. Mild conductive hearing loss in the right ear ⊘
Correct. The audiogram shows mild conductive hearing loss in the right ear. It is mild at 25–39 dB hearing loss and conductive as high-frequency hearing is relatively preserved and bone conduction (same for both ears) is normal.

B. Mild sensorineural hearing loss in the right ear
The bone conduction is unaffected.

C. Mixed hearing loss in the right ear
The bone conduction is unaffected.

D. Moderate sensorineural hearing loss in the right ear
Moderate hearing loss requires a loss of 40–69 dB.

E. Severe conductive hearing loss in the right ear
Severe hearing loss requires a loss of 70–94 dB. Hearing loss is profound if greater than 95 dB.

4.7

A. Mild conductive hearing loss in both ears
Mild hearing loss would show a reduction in hearing of 25–39 dB and bone conduction would be spared.

B. Mild sensorineural hearing loss in both ears
Mild hearing loss would show a reduction in hearing of 25–39 dB.

C. Mixed hearing loss in both ears
There would be a bigger air–bone gap.

D. Severe conductive hearing loss in both ears
Bone conduction here is equally affected.

E. Severe sensorineural hearing loss in both ears ⊘
Correct. Severe sensorineural loss in both ears. The hearing loss is severe (70–94 dB) to profound (>95 dB) and sensorineural, as there is no significant air–bone gap.

4.8

A. Cataract ⊘
Correct. This picture (Fig. 4.3) shows a white or milky coloured object in the pupil. This is due to opacification of the lens (congenital cataract). The red reflex would be absent.

B. Conjunctivitis
Conjunctivitis would present with normal development and inflamed conjunctivae.

C. Corneal trauma
Corneal trauma would be difficult to see without fluorescein eye drops.

D. Retinopathy of prematurity
Retinopathy of prematurity is increased vascularization of the retina, which may be associated with excessive oxygen therapy in premature infants. There may be loss of red reflex on ophthalmology, but the lesion is at the back and not the front of the eye.

E. Vitamin A deficiency
Vitamin A deficiency is an important cause of blindness in developing countries. It presents at an older age.

Answers: Extended Matching

4.9.1

F. CT or MRI scan of the brain
Clarissa has spastic hemiplegic cerebral palsy. She has delayed motor milestones, and a preference for using her left side from an earlier age than expected. In most instances a MRI scan would be performed rather than a CT scan, but the family may have to wait a little longer for this to be undertaken and it will require sedation.

4.9.2

B. Chromosome karyotype
Geoffrey is likely to have Down syndrome, trisomy 21. See Box 9.1 and Fig. 9.2. This can be confirmed with a karyotype or DNA FISH analysis. The latter has the advantage of being quicker and results can be available in 1–2 days. The main disadvantage of FISH analysis compared with karyotyping is that it gives less information about all of the chromosomes being studied. For example, a typical prenatal FISH test will tell you how many of the number 13, 18, 21, X and Y chromosomes are present (i.e., whether there are two copies or three) but will not give you any information about any of the other chromosomes or any information about the actual structure of chromosomes. Therefore a karyotype will be required for counselling. By 10 months and with the clinical features listed, a diagnosis of Down syndrome is highly likely and therefore it makes more sense to explain this to the family and arrange a chromosome karyotype.

4.9.3

C. Congenital infection screen
This infant has features of a congenital infection, including growth restriction, anaemia, microcephaly and hepatosplenomegaly. If he is confirmed to have congenital cytomegalovirus infection, then treatment with ganciclovir would be indicated as this has been shown to improve outcomes.

4.9.4

H. EEG
Dorcus is described as having infantile spasms. These typically appear as rapid extensions or flexions (salaam spasms). Her milestones have regressed. An EEG is required to identify hypsarrhythmia. See Table 29.1 and Fig. 29.3 in Illustrated Textbook of Paediatrics.

4.9.5

E. Creatine kinase
He may have Duchenne muscular dystrophy or one of the wide range of muscular dystrophies. Checking his creatine kinase would be the initial investigation as it is raised in muscular dystrophies. See Fig. 29.5 in Illustrated Textbook of Paediatrics.

4.10.1
E. Spastic quadriplegia
There is stiffness, hyperreflexia, and persistence of primitive reflexes. He has quadriplegia as all four limbs are affected, with the arms severely affected. Refer to Fig. 4.5 in Illustrated Textbook of Paediatrics.

4.10.2
A. Dyskinetic
In this instance, caused by kernicterus because of his severe early jaundice. He has dystonic movements and muscle spasms.

4.10.3
C. Spastic diplegia
Hassan's lower limbs are much more affected than his upper limbs; his feet are extended from markedly increased tone, causing him to walk on tiptoes, which also causes his legs to cross when he is lifted up, i.e. 'scissoring'.

4.10.4
D. Spastic hemiplegia
Alan has a right hemiplegia.

4.10.5
B: Ataxic
He is ataxic. Most cases are genetically determined and this is a relatively rare sub-type.

4.11.1
C. Paediatrician
She requires detailed assessment and investigation and management of her medical problems as well as coordination of input from therapists and other agencies. This requires specialist expertise and the experience of a paediatrician will be required.

4.11.2
H. Speech and language therapist
A speech and language therapist will assist with oro-motor coordination to establish feeding. In some centres a dietician would provide this support, or work closely with the speech and language therapist.

4.11.3
A. Dietician
The most common cause of faltering growth is inadequate calorie intake and dietician involvement is invaluable.

4.11.4
E. Psychologist
An educational psychologist will provide cognitive testing and advice on education and behaviour management. This can be helpful in obtaining the best outcomes.

4.11.5
D. Physiotherapist and occupational therapist
Physiotherapist, usually in conjunction with occupational therapist, assist with balance and mobility problems, prevention of contractures and scoliosis and advise on use of mobility aids and orthoses.

4.11.6
H. Speech and language therapist
A hearing test first is always required but if there is no hearing impairment, referral to speech and language therapy team will be indicated.

4.11.7
B. Occupational therapist
An occupational therapist would assess home suitability and whether additional aids are required. A social worker may be needed if financial assistance is required.

4.11.8
G. Specialist health visitor
A healthcare professional should visit the family home to ensure that it is safe and to offer the family advice and support that may be required. In this case a specialist health visitor would be the most appropriate professional.

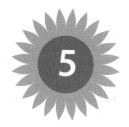

Care of the sick child and young person

Questions: Single Best Answer

5.1

Molly is 18 months old and needs to be admitted to the paediatric ward in the district hospital. There is one paediatric ward in the hospital. Her mother is concerned whether they will be geared to caring for such a young child.

What is the most common age for children to be admitted to hospital?

Select one answer only.

A. Less than 1 year
B. 1–3 years
C. 3–5 years
D. 5–10 years
E. 10–16 years

5.2

Rhys is a 4-year-old boy from Wales who is referred acutely to the paediatric team as he has developed pneumonia. He has also had increasing weakness in his legs. He has been admitted to the ward. Investigations reveal he has Duchenne muscular dystrophy.

Who is the most appropriate person to inform the parents about his diagnosis?

Select one answer only.

A. General practitioner
B. Junior doctor
C. Nurse looking after patient
D. Senior doctor
E. Sister on ward

5.3

Daniel is a 15-year-old boy who went to see his general practitioner as he has been tired and not 'quite right' for the last 2 months. The general practitioner obtained a full blood count to see if he was anaemic. The haematology laboratory phone you, a newly qualified doctor, at 6 PM in the hospital saying they have received a full blood count on Daniel and his white cells are 200 × 10⁹/L and that there are blast cells. You ring Daniel's parents at home and tell them they need to come to the oncology ward at the hospital as the results of his blood tests are abnormal. They ask you what the abnormalities are and you tell them you will explain more when they come in. You ring the consultant who says he will come to the hospital to speak to the parents. When the parents arrive you ask them to wait 20 minutes until the consultant arrives and he will explain more.

What is least ideal about the situation?

Select one answer only.

A. The family had to wait for the consultant, so you should have told them the diagnosis
B. You asked the family to come to an oncology ward rather than the paediatric assessment unit
C. You did not answer the parent's questions on the phone. You should have told them the diagnosis
D. You have asked Daniel to come out of hours rather than the following morning
E. You have told the parents over the phone the blood test was abnormal rather than in person

Questions: Extended Matching

5.4

For each of the scenarios below select the most appropriate way to administer the medication required from the list (A–I) below. Each option may be used once, more than once, or not at all.

A. Inhaled via large-volume spacer device
B. Intradermal
C. Intramuscular
D. Intravenous
E. Liquid
F. Nebulized
G. Subcutaneous
H. Tablets
I. Topical

5.4.1
Noel is a 7-day-old baby who is admitted to hospital with a fever. He is feeding 3–4-hourly from the breast and has no obvious source for his fever. He was born by vaginal delivery following a normal pregnancy.

5.4.2
Luke is a 3-year-old boy who is seen in the paediatric assessment unit. He is eating and drinking adequately. He has no other medical history and is not on any medications. He has a fever, which is associated with tachypnoea and crepitations at the right base. His oxygen saturation is 96% in air.

5.4.3
Mark is a 15-year-old boy who is seen in the emergency department with an exacerbation of wheeze. He is able to speak in short sentences but has an oxygen requirement and needs to be given salbutamol.

5.4.4
A mother has just given birth to a baby girl in a hospital in England. The midwife wants to give her vitamin K.

5.4.5
Xu-Li is a 1-year-old with significant eczema (Fig. 5.1). She has no other medical problems and is not on any medication. You decide to prescribe medication.

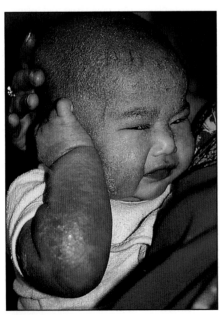

Figure 5.1

5.5
Each of the children listed below is in pain. Select the most appropriate next step in their pain management from the list (A–K) below. Each option may be used once, more than once, or not at all.

A. Distraction
B. Epidural analgesia
C. Inhalation of nitrous oxide
D. Intranasal diamorphine
E. Intravenous morphine via a nurse-controlled pump
F. Intravenous patient-controlled analgesia with morphine
G. Regular oral long-acting morphine with rapid action oramorph for breakthrough pain
H. Regular oral nonsteroidal anti-inflammatory drug (NSAID)
I. Regular oral paracetamol
J. Regular oral weak opioid, e.g. codeine
K. Topical anaesthetic

5.5.1
Charlie is a 13-month-old boy who is attending the community centre to receive his measles, mumps, and rubella vaccination. He has no medical problems, has no allergies, and is not currently on any medication.

5.5.2
Victoria is 6 months old. She attends the outpatient department for a blood test.

5.5.3
Fiona is 3 years old. She has come from her home in Northern Ireland to England to have a liver transplant. She is day 1 postoperative.

5.5.4
Jake is 3 years old. He has had a hernia repair and has just come back to the ward. You are asked to write-up some pain relief by the nurses.

5.5.5
Noah is a 7-year-old boy. He attends the Accident and Emergency department in severe pain. He has been involved in a road traffic accident and has a compound fracture of his femur. He has had several episodes of vomiting. He is extremely agitated. He has no intravenous access.

5.5.6
Zac is a 10-year-old boy who was diagnosed with Ewing sarcoma. He has severe pain from metastatic disease, which is unresponsive to therapy. You ask the palliative care team to help with his management as the medications are insufficient. You have tried regular, high-dose paracetamol without success. He has acute kidney injury secondary to his chemotherapy. He has no allergies.

5.5.7
Achille is a 13-year-old black African boy who has sickle cell disease. He presents with pain in his left leg. He has already taken paracetamol without effect. He has no other medical problems and has no allergies.

5.6
Choose from the options which best describes the reason for the doctor's actions in managing Tolla, an 11-year-old girl who has recently arrived in the UK with her mother. They are originally from Uganda. Tolla has been admitted to the paediatric ward with a chest infection. Her mother is HIV (Human immunodeficiency virus) positive but has not told any of her family members. Her husband, Tolla's father, died of an acquired immune deficiency syndrome-related illness 6 months ago. Tolla has been tested for HIV and her test result has come back positive. Her mother does not wish her to be told, as she is still very upset about the death of Tolla's father.

Each option [A–H] may be used once, more than once, or not at all.

A. Autonomy
B. Beneficence
C. Duty
D. Justice
E. Non-maleficence
F. Rights
G. Truth-telling
H. Utility

5.6.1
As Tolla's doctor you feel she should be told she is HIV positive, as you will be able to offer her more support and coping strategies if she knows more about her diagnosis.

5.6.2
As Tolla's doctor you feel she should not be told the diagnosis as this will potentially expose her and her family to more harm due to the stigma attached to having HIV. The knowledge that she is HIV positive may also affect her self-esteem.

5.6.3
As Tolla's doctor you feel she has a right to be involved in her own treatment and therefore should be told she is HIV positive.

5.6.4
Her mother has asked you to tell her the HIV test is negative and as the doctor you do not feel this is ethically right.

5.6.5
The hospital manager has asked you not to start antiretroviral therapy as the family do not have legal status to stay in the UK and cannot afford the medication. You start the therapy against this advice.

Answers: Single Best Answer

5.1
A. Less than 1 year ⊘
Correct. The most common age is infants less than 1 year. Most medical admissions are emergencies in children under 5 years of age, whereas surgical admissions peak at 5 years of age, one-third of which are elective.

5.2
A. General practitioner
In some instances, the general practitioner will know the family well and may be a great support. However, they are unlikely to have looked after a child with Duchenne muscular dystrophy before and may not be able to answer all the family's questions.

B. Junior doctor
Junior doctors often offer great support and empathy to families, but families prefer serious or complex information to be delivered by a senior doctor. However, as junior doctors (and nurses) are likely to be questioned by parents before being seen by a senior doctor, it can be difficult to avoid revealing information best reserved for an interview with the most appropriate professionals and members of the family being present.

C. Nurse looking after patient
The nurse looking after a patient will be able to provide support to the family and can often help the family with questions after the diagnosis has been given to them.

D. Senior doctor ⊘
Correct. Parents say that they would prefer a senior doctor, in the presence of a nurse, to communicate serious or complex information to them.

E. Sister on ward
May provide considerable support to the medical and nursing teams and families but most parents report that they would prefer serious or complex information to be communicated by a senior doctor.

5.3
A. The family had to wait for the consultant, so you should have told them the diagnosis
Breaking bad news is always difficult and should be done by a senior doctor. A 20-minute wait is not a good reason to tell them the diagnosis.

B. You asked the family to come to an oncology ward rather than the paediatric assessment unit ⊘
Correct. By telling them to come to an oncology ward you are telling them Daniel has cancer without actually explaining his diagnosis properly.

C. You did not answer the parent's questions on the phone. You should have told them the diagnosis
You need to give some explanation of why Daniel should come back to hospital but it is better to break the bad news in person rather than over the phone.

D. You have asked Daniel to come out of hours rather than the following morning
Daniel needs to come to hospital as soon as possible because of the high white cell count, so the family needed to come out of hours rather than waiting until morning.

E. You have told the parents over the phone the blood test was abnormal rather than in person
You need to give some explanation of why Daniel should come back to hospital.

Answers: Extended Matching

5.4.1
D. Intravenous
In acutely ill neonates and infants, drugs are given intravenously to ensure reliable and adequate blood and tissue concentrations. Fever without a source in this age group is an indication for a septic screen and starting intravenous antibiotics. With oral formulations, intake cannot be guaranteed and absorption is unpredictable as it is affected by gastric emptying and acidity, gut motility and the effects of milk in the stomach.

5.4.2
E. Liquid
He has a community-acquired pneumonia but is systemically well. For the treatment of uncomplicated pneumonia, oral therapy is as good as intravenous treatment. He could be given antibiotics in liquid form; he is too young to take tablets. If he was systemically unwell and had signs of a pleural effusion or empyema, intravenous therapy would be indicated. (See the PIVOT study for more details. Available at: http://www.ncbi.nlm.nih.gov/pmc/articles/PMC2094276/.)

5.4.3
F. Nebulized
Nebulized treatment should be given when there is an oxygen requirement, as it is not possible to administer supplemental oxygen whilst treatment is given by inhaler and large-volume spacer.

If he did not have an oxygen requirement, the best way to deliver the salbutamol is a metered-dose inhaler with a spacer, as this is as effective without the extra cost of a nebulizer or the increased risk of paradoxical desaturation. He should also be given oral steroids. (See: http://openaccess.sgul.ac.uk/2699/1/CD000052.pdf.)

5.4.4
C. Intramuscular
Intramuscular (IM) vitamin K is recommended for all infants to prevent haemorrhagic disease of the newborn. Parents may request oral vitamin K as an alternative; although care should be taken to identify why. Some poor evidence synthesis in the 1990s raised questions about IM vitamin K and long-term risk of childhood leukaemia – this was unsubstantiated and IM vitamin K is now recommended. As oral absorption is variable, three doses are needed orally over the first 4 weeks of life to achieve adequate liver storage, but protection cannot be guaranteed. [See: http://evidencebasedbirth.com/evidence-for-the -vitamin-k-shot-in-newborns/ for a very helpful (if somewhat US centric) description of why IM vitamin K is preferable to oral vitamin K and a discussion of the evidence concerning childhood leukaemia.]

5.4.5
I. Topical
Most medication for eczema is topical. Emollients are the first line of therapy (if it is dry, then wet it). These should be administered topically and applied regularly. The skin needs to be kept moist to prevent scratching.
A good way of assessing how often it is applied is to ask how quickly the pot of emollient was finished.

5.5.1
A. Distraction
Distraction is very effective for reducing pain and distress during minor procedures.

5.5.2
K. Topical anaesthetic
Distraction would also be useful but applying some topical anaesthetic cream is effective at preventing pain from a blood test.

5.5.3
E. Intravenous morphine via a nurse-controlled pump
Liver transplantation is a major operation and the child would experience considerable pain. At 3 years of age she is too young for a patient-controlled pump.

5.5.4
I. Regular oral paracetamol
Paracetamol is a useful analgesic especially if given regularly. Nonsteroidal anti-inflammatory drugs (NSAIDs) should be given as second line; ibuprofen can be helpful if there is no contra-indication. Morphine would not normally be required after a hernia repair.

5.5.5
D. Intranasal diamorphine
The oral and intravenous routes are not available in this situation. Inhalation of nitrous oxide is also an effective analgesia when the oral or intravenous route is not available. However, the child needs to cooperate to be able to use it effectively. Most 7-year-olds will not find it particularly helpful unless they already know how to use it. A child in severe pain who is upset will find it very difficult to learn a new skill.

5.5.6
G. Regular oral long-acting morphine with rapid action oramorph for breakthrough pain
Pain from metastatic disease can be very severe. NSAIDs should be avoided in renal failure.

5.5.7
H. NSAID
Achille needs a regular NSAID. Sickle cell crises can be very painful and there may be a need to escalate to an oral opioid medication. However, opioid dependence can become a problem in patients with sickle cell disease.

5.6.1
B. Beneficence
The child's interest is paramount. In the UK, this is enshrined in the Children Act 1989 and the UN Convention on the Rights of the Child. Beneficence is the positive obligation to do good (this principle has been part of medical ethics since the Hippocratic Oath).

5.6.2
E. Non-maleficence
Do no harm (psychological and/or physical). This principle has been part of medical ethics since the Hippocratic Oath.

5.6.3
A. Autonomy
Respect for individuals' rights to make informed and thought-out decisions for themselves in accordance with their capabilities.

5.6.4
G. Truth telling
This and confidentiality are important aspects of autonomy that support trust, essential in the doctor–patient relationship.

5.6.5
C. Duty
Duty is the moral obligation to act irrespective of the consequences in accordance with moral laws, which are universal, apply equally to all, and which respect persons as autonomous beings. There is also a degree of justice to this situation.

Paediatric emergencies

6.1

The paediatric team is resuscitating a 3-month-old boy who is in pulseless electrical activity. He was discovered to be blue and lifeless when his parents went to wake him in the morning. The airway has been secured and despite bag valve mask ventilation the child remains blue. Cardiac compressions are given.

Where is the most appropriate position on the chest (Fig. 6.1) to do cardiac compressions?

Select one answer only.

A. A
B. B
C. C
D. None of the above
E. All of the above

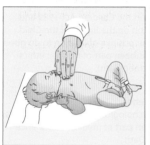
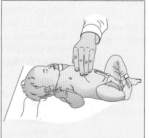
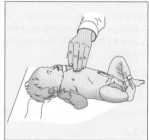

| A | B | C |

Figure 6.1

6.2

You are in the Acute Assessment Unit and see David, a 15-month-old boy, who has a fever of 38.5°C. He has had a runny nose, cough and a fever for 3 days. Since this morning he has slept and has been difficult to wake. His heart rate is raised. He has a rash (Fig. 6.2) scattered over his legs which does not disappear with pressure.

Which of the following is the most likely diagnosis?

Select one answer only.

A. Acute lymphoblastic leukaemia
B. Henoch–Schönlein purpura
C. Immune thrombocytopenia
D. Non-accidental injury
E. Septicaemia

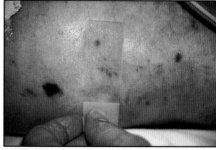

Figure 6.2

6.3

A 3-year-old boy who is unconscious arrives in the Emergency Department. You manage his airway, breathing and circulation. His blood glucose is normal. On examination you note his pupils are as in Fig. 6.3. His temperature and other vital signs are otherwise normal.

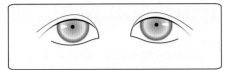

Figure 6.3

What is the most likely cause?

Select one answer only.

A. Third nerve lesion
B. Severe hypoxia
C. Hypothermia
D. Tentorial herniation
E. Opiate poisoning

6.4

You are called to see a 3-year-old boy with a high fever. The nurse is worried that he is very sleepy. As you walk into the resuscitation room he makes no spontaneous response. You try calling his name but he makes no response. On stimulation, his eyes open, he cries and he raises his hand and pushes your hand away.

What is this child's Glasgow Coma Score (GCS)?

Select one answer only.

A. 8
B. 9
C. 10
D. 11
E. 12

6.5

Ryan, aged 10 months, is rushed to the children's emergency department after being found submerged in the bath. His mother runs screaming into the department saying 'Help my baby, please'.

Which is the next most appropriate step?

Select one answer only.

A. Commence chest compressions in a ratio of 15:2
B. If the child is not breathing, commence bag and mask ventilation
C. Place the child onto the examination couch and put his head into the neutral position

D. Remove wet clothing/towels and dry the baby vigorously
E. Stimulate the baby and shout for help

6.6

Mohammed, aged 8 months, has been vomiting and off his feeds for 2 days. Initially, he had episodes of crying uncontrollably, drawing his legs up into his abdomen as if in pain, and appeared fractious. His mother gave him some oral rehydration solution, but his vomiting continued and he has become lethargic. On admission to hospital he is in shock.

What is the most likely diagnosis?

Select one answer only.

A. Gastroenteritis
B. Intussusception
C. Malrotation and volvulus
D. Meckel diverticulum
E. Strangulated hernia

6.7

Mohammed, aged 8 months, presented with the clinical scenario described in question 6.7. He weighs 8 kg. He needs a bolus of normal saline 0.9% to treat his shock.

What volume of fluid would you give initially?

Select one answer only.

A. 40 ml
B. 160 ml
C. 320 ml
D. 680 ml
E. 800 ml

6.8

Mohammed, aged 8 months, has presented with the clinical scenario described in Questions 6.6 and 6.7. He has received the fluid bolus of normal saline 0.9%, which has improved his condition. From his presentation you suspect he is 10% dehydrated. You receive his laboratory results, which reveal a plasma sodium of 138 mmol/L (within the normal range). His continuing fluid loss from vomiting is small and can be ignored.

What is Mohammed's total fluid requirement for the initial 24 hours? He weighs 8 kg.

Select one answer only.

A. 160 ml
B. 320 ml
C. 800 ml
D. 880 ml
E. 1600 ml

6.9

You are called to the resuscitation room where there is a 6-year-old child who has arrived by ambulance. The child has been having a generalized seizure for 15 minutes. The ambulance crew gave a dose of buccal midazolam 5 minutes ago. The emergency doctor has maintained the airway and has applied oxygen. His capillary refill time is less than 2 seconds and his heart rate 120 beats/min.

What is the next most appropriate management step?

Select one answer only.

A. Administer further anticonvulsant
B. Check blood glucose level
C. Gain intravenous access
D. Request senior review
E. Start bag and valve mask ventilation

6.10

Seb, a 2-year-old boy, was at his cousin's birthday party. His mother noticed that he has suddenly developed a widespread urticarial rash and has also become flushed in the face. His vital signs are normal and he has no respiratory compromise.

Which medication would you give?

Select one answer only.

A. Intramuscular adrenaline
B. Intramuscular antihistamine
C. Intravenous hydrocortisone
D. Oral antihistamine
E. Oral corticosteroid

6.11

Jenny, a 3-year-old girl, was at a village fete. She suddenly developed swollen cheeks and lips and a widespread urticarial rash. She is rushed to the nearby general practice surgery, where it is noted that her breathing is very noisy. She is distressed and frightened. On auscultation she has widespread wheeze.

Which medication would you give first?

A. Intramuscular adrenaline
E. Intramuscular antihistamine
C. Intravenous hydrocortisone
D. Oral antihistamine
B. Oral corticosteroid

6.12

There has been a dramatic decline in the incidence of sudden infant death syndrome in the UK.

Which of the following is the single most important factor responsible for this decline?

A. Feet to foot of cot
B. Keeping baby in parent's room until 6 months of age
C. Keeping room cool to prevent overheating
D. Parents not smoking in the same room as infant
E. Supine sleeping

Questions: Extended Matching

6.13

For each of the following patients seen in the emergency department select the most appropriate next step in the management plan from the following list (A–L). Each option may be used once, more than once, or not at all.

A. Airway opening manoeuvres
B. Bag and mask ventilation
C. Check blood glucose
D. Check conscious level [alert, voice, pain, unresponsive (AVPU)]
E. Check pupils
F. Commence cardiac compressions using both hands, one hand on top of the other
G. Commence cardiac compressions using the encircling method
H. Commence cardiac compressions using one hand on the sternum
I. High-flow oxygen therapy
J. Intravenous access
K. Intravenous fluid
L. Secondary survey

6.13.1

Nathaniel, a 4-year-old boy, is brought to hospital with shortness of breath. He is able to talk but has oxygen saturation of 90%. His capillary refill time is less than 2 seconds.

6.13.2

Kelsey, a 2-year-old girl, is found unconscious in the garden. When she is bought into the resuscitation room she is gasping and moaning.

6.13.3

Ahmed, aged 2 months, is found by his mother to be pale and floppy in his cot. The paramedics are giving bag and valve mask ventilation when he arrives in the resuscitation room and his chest is moving well. His heart rate is 40 beats/min.

6.13.4

Daniel, age 10 years, has diabetes mellitus and has been playing football at his friend's house. He has been brought to the emergency department as he has become confused and is sweaty. He walks into the department.

6.13.5

Aisha, a 3-year-old girl, is bought to hospital by the paramedics as she has had a seizure. She is receiving high-flow oxygen, her breathing is regular, and the cardiac monitor shows a heart rate of 100 beats/min. She is unresponsive to painful stimuli, as she does not flinch when her blood glucose is checked.

Answers: Single Best Answer

6.1
B. B ⊘
Correct. In infants the heart is lower in relation to the external landmarks than in older children or adults. The area of compression over the sternum should be one finger breadth below an imaginary line between the nipples.

6.2
A. Acute lymphoblastic leukaemia
This is a short history of the child being unwell. In acute lymphoblastic leukaemia you would expect a longer history and other characteristic clinical features.

B. Henoch–Schönlein purpura
The purpuric rash is localized to the legs and buttocks, Henoch–Schönlein purpura is associated with abdominal pain and joint pain but not with fever and being severely ill.

C. Immune thrombocytopenia
With immune thrombocytopenia the children are usually well.

D. Non-accidental injury
Non-accidental injury is not suggested by this acute febrile illness.

E. Septicaemia ⊘
Correct. He has a purpuric rash, with lesions of variable size. In a febrile child, meningococcal septicaemia is most likely. This is not invariably accompanied by meningitis.

6.3
A. Third nerve lesion
Third nerve lesions and tentorial herniation would cause a unilaterally dilated pupil.

B. Severe hypoxia
Severe hypoxia would cause dilated pupils.

C. Hypothermia
With hypothermia the child's temperature would be low and it causes dilated pupils.

D. Tentorial herniation
Third nerve lesions and tentorial herniation would cause a unilaterally dilated pupil.

E. Opiate poisoning ⊘
Correct. Bilateral, pinpoint pupils (as in Fig. 6.3) with coma can be caused by a pontine lesion or opiate poisoning. Opiate poisoning may occur in homes with substance abusers or adults on methadone.

6.4
A. 8
The Glasgow Coma Scale is shown in Table 6.1 below. This child is scoring more than 8 as

pushing a hand away suggests localization. Remember, the lowest possible score in each domain is 1 (rather than 0).

B. 9 ⊘
Correct. The Glasgow Coma Scale is made up of three parts. *Best motor response* (a score of 1–6 is possible); *Best verbal response* (a score of 1–5 is possible) and *Best eye opening* (1–4 is possible). Here the child scores 5 for best motor response (localizes pain) and 2 each for best verbal and best eye response.

C. 10
The verbal score here would have been higher if the child had responded with vocal sounds or words and for eye opening if he had responded to sounds rather than pain.

D. 11
Remember that there is a separate scoring system for children under 4 years of age.

E. 12
This child is only responsive to pain. Using the AVPU (alert, voice, pain, unresponsive) scoring system, a score of P usually corresponds to a GCS of 8 or 9.

6.5
A. Commence chest compressions in a ratio of 15:2
Chest compressions may be required but this is further down the resuscitation algorithm.

B. If the child is not breathing, commence bag and mask ventilation
This is done after stimulating the child, shouting for help and opening the airway.

C. Place the child onto the examination couch and put his head into the neutral position
This will need to be done, but is not the first step.

D. Remove wet clothing/towels and dry the baby vigorously
Drying is an essential first step in a newborn infant but not the first thing to do here.

E. Stimulate the baby and shout for help ⊘
Correct. All resuscitation algorithms ensure that the patient is assessed in a sequential manner, adopting an Airway, Breathing and Circulation approach. The paediatric life support algorithm states that you: 1. Check safety (not strictly necessary within hospital), stimulate and shout for help. Calling for help early on in these situations is paramount as you need many people for resuscitation.

6.6
A. Gastroenteritis
Less likely, because episodes of crying uncontrollably with drawing of legs up into his

Table 6.1 Glasgow Coma Scale, incorporating Children's Coma Scale

	Glasgow Coma Scale (4–15 years)	Children's Coma Scale (<4 years)	
	Response	Response	Score
Eye opening	Spontaneous	Spontaneous	4
	To sound	To sound	3
	To pressure	To pain	2
	None	No response	1
Best motor response	Obeys commands	Obeys commands	6
	Localizes pain	Localizes pain	5
	Normal flexion	Flexion to pain	4
	Abnormal flexion	Abnormal flexion (decorticate posture)	3
	Extension	Abnormal extension (decerebrate posture)	2
	No response	No response	1
Best verbal response	Oriented	Talks normally, interacts	5
	Confused	Words	4
	Words	Vocal sounds	3
	Sounds	Cries	2
	No response	No response	1

A score of <8 out of 15 means that the child's airway is at risk and will need to be maintained by a manoeuvre or adjunct.

abdomen as if in pain are characteristic of intussusception.

B. Intussusception ⊘
Correct. Intussusception is the most likely cause of the pain and shock. Although this could be a strangulated hernia, this should be evident on clinical examination. Follow an Airway, Breathing, Circulation approach, get senior help and speak to the radiologist. The diagnosis might be obvious on ultrasound.

C. Malrotation and volvulus
Less likely, because episodes of crying uncontrollably with drawing of legs up into his abdomen as if in pain are characteristic of intussusception. Bile-stained vomiting is often present in malrotation. However, the diagnosis must be considered.

D. Meckel diverticulum
Meckel diverticulum tends to present with bleeding per rectum as well as abdominal pain. Blood loss is rarely so severe to result in shock.

E. Strangulated hernia
Although this could be a strangulated hernia, this should be evident on clinical examination.

6.7
B. 160 ml ⊘
Correct. This is 20 ml/kg initially, repeated as necessary. See Fig. 6.9 in Illustrated Textbook of

Paediatrics for initial fluid resuscitation in shock. In trauma or diabetic ketoacidosis smaller aliquots are given.

6.8
E. 1600 ml ⊘
Correct. Mohammed's fluid requirement is calculated by adding
- Deficit: 10% of 8 kg = 800 ml
- Maintenance: 100 ml/kg per 24 hours = 800 ml
- Continuing losses: 0 ml

Total = 1600 ml
See Table 6.1 in Illustrated Textbook of Paediatrics for maintenance fluid requirements at different weights.

6.9
A. Administer further anticonvulsant
After 10 minutes it is recommended to give a further dose of an anticonvulsant if still having a seizure.

B. Check blood glucose level ⊘
Correct. This is the most appropriate next step as, if the patient is hypoglycaemic, the only treatment to stop the seizure would be to administer glucose. Ideally, intravenous glucose will be given but if access is not achieved, then glucose gel buccally.

C. Gain intravenous access
It is difficult to do this whilst the child is having a seizure. It can be very helpful but there are more important treatment steps. This is often done at the same time by other team members.

D. Request senior review
It is important to make an ABC plus *don't ever forget glucose* (ABCDEFG) assessment yourself before seeking senior review.

E. Start bag and valve mask ventilation
Although it can be difficult to assess breathing in a child with seizures, it is usually sufficient to administer oxygen unless breathing stops completely. This can occur after benzodiazepine therapy but is uncommon after a single dose.

6.10
A. Intramuscular adrenaline
This is not needed as there is no respiratory compromise.

B. Intramuscular antihistamine
This is not indicated as it is painful to administer and the child is able to take oral medicines, as there is no respiratory compromise.

C. Intravenous hydrocortisone
This is not needed as this is a mild allergic reaction and there is no respiratory compromise.

D. Oral antihistamine ⊘
Correct. In children, the most common causes of acute food allergy are ingestion or contact with nuts, egg, milk or seafood. Urticaria and facial swelling are mild reactions. Immediate management is with an oral antihistamine (e.g., chlorphenamine) and observation over 2 hours for possible complications.

E. Oral corticosteroid
This is not needed as this is a mild allergic reaction and there is no respiratory compromise. The condition should respond to oral antihistamine.

6.11
A. Intramuscular adrenaline ⊘
Correct. This child has anaphylaxis, which is life threatening as she has both upper airway obstruction (noisy breathing) and bronchoconstriction (wheeze). Either of these on their own or any signs of shock would be enough to constitute a diagnosis of anaphylaxis. Priority is to manage the airway and give oxygen via a non-rebreathe mask. The first medication to give would be intramuscular adrenaline.

E. Intramuscular antihistamine
This would make the situation worse, as it is painful and will not directly treat the upper airway obstruction.

C. Intravenous hydrocortisone
This should only be given after immediate treatment of the upper airway obstruction with intramuscular adrenaline. Also, her upper airway obstruction may be further compromised by the distress of establishing an intravenous cannula. It takes about 6 hours to have optimal effect.

D. Oral antihistamine
Antihistamine alone will be slow to work and rapid treatment is required.

B. Oral corticosteroid
This child has upper airway obstruction so is unlikely to be able to take oral medications and oral steroids would take too long to work.

6.12
E. Supine sleeping ⊘
Correct. All the answers have helped reduce the risk of sudden infant death syndrome, but the single most important factor is putting babies to sleep on their backs.

Answers: Extended Matching

6.13.1
I. High-flow oxygen therapy
He has a patent airway as he is able to talk. His oxygen saturation is low, so oxygen needs to be given. This will improve co-operation and reduce anxiety.

6.13.2
A. Airway opening manoeuvres
She is gasping and moaning, and thus needs her airway repositioning before commencing bag and valve mask ventilation.

6.13.3
G. Commence cardiac compressions using the hands encircling method
Ahmed has a heart rate of less than 40 beats/min and his airway and breathing are being managed. Therefore cardiac compressions need to be started. The most effective way in this age group is the hand encircling technique. The main disadvantage of this technique is that it requires at least two rescuers to provide effective, timely basic life support.

6.13.4
C. Blood glucose
The clinical features suggest hypoglycaemia.

6.13.5
E. Check pupils
Her pupils need checking as her airway, breathing, circulation, and conscious level have already been checked.

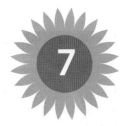

Accidents and poisoning

Questions: Single Best Answer

7.1
What is the most common cause of death in children aged 1 year to 14 years in the UK?

Select one answer only.

A. Accidents
B. Congenital heart disease
C. Infectious disease
D. Malignant disease
E. Respiratory disease

7.2
Hamim, a boy aged 3 years, fell 3 metres from a first-floor balcony on to a concrete path. He presents to the Emergency Department with his parents who are concerned that he has vomited several times since the episode. After the fall he immediately cried out in pain, but appeared to be all right. His mother reports that he did not lose consciousness. On examination he is found to be fully conscious but has a large bruise over the left parietal region. There are neither focal neurological signs nor any other injuries. His heart rate is 110 beats/min, his respiratory rate is 25 breaths/min and his blood pressure is 90/50 mmHg.

Which of the following would be the most worrying additional clinical sign?

Select one answer only.

A. A black eye (bruising around left eye)
B. A fractured nose with deviated septum
C. A runny nose
D. A temperature of 38.2°C
E. Further enlargement of the parietal bruising

7.3
Hamim (as outlined in Question 7.2) has a lateral skull X-ray taken (Fig. 7.1).

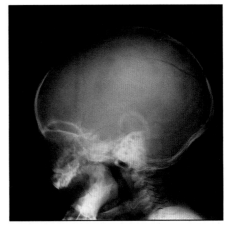

Figure 7.1

What does the X-ray show?

Select one answer only.

A. Frontal bone fracture
B. No abnormalities shown
C. Occipital bone fracture
D. Parietal bone fracture
E. Temporal bone fracture

7.4
Hamim (as outlined in Question 7.3) is admitted to hospital for a period of observation.

Eight hours after admission, the nurses note a change in his level of consciousness. He is now responsive only to painful stimuli; his left pupil is dilated although still responsive to light. His airway, breathing and circulation are satisfactory. A CT scan (Fig. 7.2) shows that there is a haemorrhage and a skull fracture. He is stabilized in the resuscitation room.

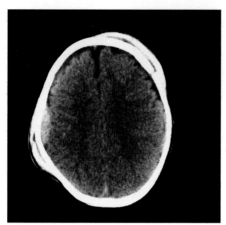

Figure 7.2

Which of the following is the most appropriate next step in his management?

Select one answer only.

A. Clotting studies
B. EEG
C. Neurosurgical referral
D. Ophthalmology opinion
E. Skeletal survey

7.5
Louise, aged 4 years, was hit by a car in the local supermarket car park. She is brought to the Emergency Department by ambulance.

An initial assessment shows

- Airway — talking to mother
- Breathing — receiving oxygen via a rebreathing circuit, oxygen saturation 99%
- Breathing — air entry satisfactory and equal bilaterally, respiratory rate 30/min
- Circulation — pulse 160/min, blood pressure 90/50 mmHg, capillary refill time 3 seconds
- Disability — alert, but frightened and agitated, moving all four limbs

She has abrasions to her left flank and pain in her left shoulder.

What is the next intervention needed?

Select one answer only.

A. Analgesia
B. Blood glucose measurement
C. Chest X-ray
D. Intravenous access
E. Intubation and ventilation

7.6
Louise (as outlined in Question 7.5) has chest and abdominal X-rays which show fractures of the 9th and 10th ribs on the left-hand side.

What is the most important investigation to perform to establish the cause of her condition?

Select one answer only.

A. Abdominal ultrasound
B. Arrange CT head scan
C. Cervical spine X-ray
D. Full blood count
E. Serum creatinine, urea and electrolytes

7.7
Roberto is a 2.5-year-old boy. He pulled a chip pan off the cooker and has been extensively burnt. He is rushed to the nearest Children's Emergency Department. His airway, breathing and circulation are satisfactory. His burns are distributed on his body as shown in Fig. 7.3. Most of the burnt area is now blistering and mottled in colour, with a few white areas. Intravenous analgesia is given.

What is the estimated area of the burn?

Select one answer only.

A. 15%
B. 20%
C. 25%
D. 30%
E. 35%

7.8
Roberto (as outlined in Question 7.7) is much more settled following intravenous analgesia.

From the list of possible management options below, which should be undertaken first?

Select one answer only.

A. Commence intravenous 0.9% saline
B. Cover the burns with sterile dressings
C. Intravenous antibiotics
D. Intubation and artificial ventilation
E. Place affected areas in cold water

7.9
Jake is a 3-year-old boy. His brother spilt a pan of hot water over him and he has been extensively scalded. He is rushed to the nearest Emergency Department. His airway and breathing are satisfactory. He is tachycardiac, his capillary refill time is 4 seconds and he has

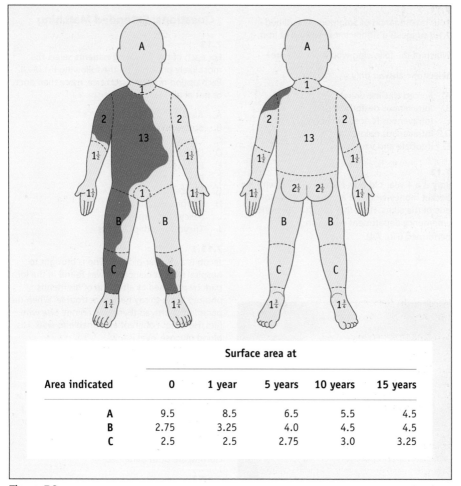

Figure 7.3

Area indicated	Surface area at				
	0	1 year	5 years	10 years	15 years
A	9.5	8.5	6.5	5.5	4.5
B	2.75	3.25	4.0	4.5	4.5
C	2.5	2.5	2.75	3.0	3.25

a low blood pressure. He has 20% burns involving his chest, abdomen, and his right arm and hand.

What is the most likely underlying cause for his shock?

Select one answer only.

A. It is secondary to the pain from his burn
B. Jake has shock due to loss of blood plasma, because of damage to his blood vessels secondary to his scald
C. Jake has shock due to loss of red blood cells, because of damage to his blood vessels secondary to his scald
D. Jake has shock due to vasodilation of his blood vessels, secondary to his scald
E. He has shock due to vasodilation of his blood vessels, secondary to infection developing in his scald

7.10

Solomon, aged 3 years, has been found eating some of his pregnant mother's iron tablets; up to 10 tablets are missing. Their general practitioner advised that he should be taken to hospital directly. On examination in the Emergency Department he is found to be talkative, with no obvious abnormalities. He has no other medical problems and is not normally on any medications.

What would be the first investigation you would perform?

Select one answer only.

A. Abdominal X-ray
B. Full blood count
C. Clotting studies
E. Liver function tests
D. Serum iron

7.11
Your investigation of Solomon (as outlined in 7.10) suggests a significant ingestion of iron.

Which of the following would you initiate?

Select one answer only.

A.   Forced alkaline diuresis
B.   Intravenous desferrioxamine
C.   Intravenous N-acetylcysteine
D.   Intravenous naloxone
E.   Intubate and ventilate

7.12
Rory is a 4-year-old boy. He was playing with his pocket money when he accidentally swallowed one of the coins. His father brings him to the emergency department where an X-ray is performed (Fig. 7.4).

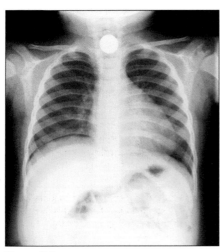

Figure 7.4

Where, anatomically, is this swallowed foreign body most likely to have lodged?

Select one answer only.

A.   Cricopharyngeus muscle
B.   Lower oesophageal sphincter
C.   Region where the aortic arch and carina overlap
D.   Thyroid cartilage
E.   Upper trachea

Questions: Extended Matching

7.13
For each of the following patients select the most likely poison from the following list (A–J). Each option may be used once, more than once, or not at all.

A.   Alcohol
B.   Button battery ingestion
C.   Cannabis
D.   Digoxin
E.   Ecstasy (MDMA)
F.   Iron
G.   Paracetamol
H.   Petroleum distillates
I.   Salicylates (aspirin)
J.   Tricyclic antidepressants

7.13.1
Jacob is a 15-year-old boy who is brought to hospital by ambulance. He was found in the local park by paramedics after one of his friends phoned them to say he was in trouble. When the paramedics arrived there was no one else with him. He is not coherent and unable to walk. His blood glucose level is low.

7.13.2
Ruby is a 15-year-old girl who attends the Emergency Department with her father as she has 'turned yellow'. When you ask her if she has taken any medicines, she says no. She is being bullied at school, which has been going on for over a year now. On examination, she is jaundiced and her liver function tests and clotting are both deranged.

7.13.3
Callum, a 15-year-old boy, is bought into the Emergency Department with his mother. She found him in his bedroom with some pills by his bed. He is disorientated and hyperventilating.

7.13.4
Syam, a 2-year-old boy, comes to the Emergency Department with his father. His mother noticed that his stools had become black. Syam lives at home with his parents, grandparents, and two siblings. Syam's mother is currently pregnant. On examination, Syam is cardiovascularly stable.

7.13.5
Adrian is a 4-year-old who has been staying with his grandmother over the weekend. He is bought to the Accident and Emergency department by his grandmother who is worried he has taken one of her heart pills. He complains of a 'funny' feeling in his chest. On examination he has an irregular heart beat and ECG reveals an arrhythmia.

Answers: Single Best Answer

7.1

A. Accidents
This is now the second most common cause of death in children aged 1 year to 14 years in the UK.

B. Congenital heart disease
This is the most common congenital malformation affecting 0.8% of liveborn children but not the most common cause of death in this age group.

C. Infectious diseases
Most common cause worldwide but not in the UK.

D. Malignant disease ⊘
Correct. Reduction in deaths from accidents, particularly in road traffic accidents, have recently made malignancy the most common cause of death in children aged 1 year to 14 years in the UK.

E. Respiratory disease
Asthma is the most common chronic disease of childhood but fortunately deaths are rare.

7.2

A. A black eye (bruising around left eye)
Black eyes (periorbital ecchymosis) are a significant sign if bilateral, as this can indicate a basal skull fracture.

B. A fractured nose with deviated septum
Parietal bruising, a fractured nose or facial laceration are all distressing, but do not suggest significant brain or skull injury.

C. A runny nose ⊘
Correct. A nasal discharge post head trauma is a significant sign. It may be leakage of cerebrospinal fluid (CSF) that can indicate a basal skull fracture. If it is CSF it will be positive for glucose on testing.

D. A temperature of 38.2°C
It is too soon for intracranial infection to be causing a fever.

E. Further enlargement of the parietal bruising
Parietal bruising, a fractured nose or facial laceration are all distressing, but do not suggest significant brain or skull injury.

7.3

D. Parietal bone fracture ⊘
Correct. A parietal fracture (Fig. 7.5) is the most common skull fracture sustained by children, whether accidental or non-accidental.

7.4

A. Clotting studies
The priority for this child is to prevent further secondary brain injury.

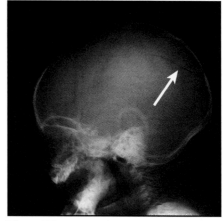

Figure 7.5

B. EEG
The priority for this child is to prevent further secondary brain injury. An EEG is not required.

C. Neurosurgical referral ⊘
Correct. This child has sustained a potentially serious head injury and now has reduced level of consciousness and focal neurological signs, which are indications to be assessed by a neurosurgical specialist. The priority for this child is to prevent further secondary brain injury.

D. Ophthalmology opinion
His abnormal pupil is caused by the intracranial lesion and not ocular pathology.

E. Skeletal survey
A skeletal survey to identify other fractures is important but the priority for this child is to prevent further secondary brain injury.

7.5

A. Analgesia
Analgesia and a blood sugar are important but not until she has some intravenous fluid.

B. Blood glucose measurement
Analgesia and a blood glucose measurement are important but not until she has some intravenous fluid.

C. Chest X-ray
A chest X-ray is needed but this comes after ABC.

D. Intravenous access ⊘
Correct. Louise has cardiovascular compromise and urgently needs fluid resuscitation. She therefore needs intravenous access.

E. Intubation and ventilation
Her airway and breathing are stable therefore the next appropriate treatment is C – circulation.

7.6
A. Abdominal ultrasound ✓
Correct. The history and signs suggest hypovolaemic shock from splenic injury. She needs an urgent abdominal ultrasound scan (FAST scan, focused abdominal sonography in trauma).

B. Arrange CT head scan
This would be indicated if there was focal neurology on secondary survey.

C. Cervical spine X-ray
Important, but clinical assessment is needed for 'clearing' a cervical spine. An experienced Emergency Department doctor will be required to guide investigation of this potential problem. For now, keep the child immobilised.

D. Full blood count
Useful, but even if anaemic it will not tell you where the blood has been lost or the volume of acute blood loss.

E. Serum creatinine, urea and electrolytes
Commonly undertaken, but rarely informative in an acute injury.

7.7
B. 20% ✓
Correct. Burns are to chest and abdomen (about 11%), right arm 2% and right leg 6%, which is 19%, i.e. approximately 20%.

7.8
A. Commence intravenous 0.9% saline ✓
Correct. There will be significant fluid loss through the burnt areas, which needs replacing.

B. Cover the burns with sterile dressings
Covering the burns is helpful but not urgent. It may help to reduce the pain experienced though.

C. Intravenous antibiotics
Intravenous antibiotics are not needed urgently.

D. Intubation and artificial ventilation
Intubation and ventilation are not required as his airway and breathing are satisfactory. It should be considered early for children with burns who have potential inhalation injury.

E. Place affected areas in cold water
Placing scalded area in cold water is useful for pain relief for small burns, but inappropriate for large burns.

7.9
A. It is secondary to the pain from his scald
His burn would be painful but this would be likely to cause a tachycardia and increase in blood pressure rather than a drop in blood pressure.

B. Jake has shock due to loss of blood plasma, because of damage to his blood vassels secondary to his scald ✓

Correct. Jake has hypovolaemic shock secondary to the loss of blood plasma. This is secondary to loss of skin integrity.

C. Jake has shock due to loss of red blood cells, because of damage to his blood vessels secondary to his scald
Jake has hypovolaemic shock secondary to the loss of blood plasma. This happens due to loss of skin integrity.

D. Jake has shock due to vasodilation of his blood vessels secondary to his scald
Jake has hypovolaemic shock secondary to the loss of blood plasma. This happens due to loss of skin integrity.

E. He has shock due to vasodilation of his blood vessels, secondary to infection developing in his scald
Though you can develop septic shock from infected burns this is likely to happen later rather than immediately.

7.10
A. Abdominal X-ray ✓
Correct. An abdominal X-ray identifies if there is a significant number of tablets in his stomach. A very useful consequence of iron showing up on X-ray!

B. Full blood count
The full blood count will be of no value at this stage.

C. Clotting studies
The clotting studies will be of no value at this stage.

D. Liver function tests
It is too soon for LFTs to become deranged.

E. Serum iron
The serum iron result will not be helpful at this stage as he will not have absorbed the medication.

7.11
A. Forced alkaline diuresis
For aspirin overdose.

B. Intravenous desferrioxamine ✓
Correct. Intravenous desferrioxamine binds with iron in the blood excreting it in urine and faeces.

C. Intravenous N-acetylcysteine
Intravenous acetylcysteine is the antidote for paracetamol poisoning.

D. Intravenous naloxone
Intravenous naloxone is the antidote for opiate poisoning.

E. Intubate and ventilate
Required if airway compromise is imminent.

7.12

A. Cricopharyngeus muscle ✓

Correct. About 70% of blunt objects that lodge in the oesophagus will do so at the cricopharyngeus muscle. Once the object reaches the stomach it is much less likely to lead to complications, though the ileocecal valve is another area that the object can lodge. The coin should be removed endoscopically.

B. Lower oesophageal sphincter
Objects tend not to get stuck here and it would appear on the chest x-ray much closer to the diaphragm if it was.

C. Region where the aortic arch and carina overlap
This would be in the mid-oesophagus.

D. Thyroid cartilage
It is too big to have passed through the larynx. Think about the size of an endotracheal tube.

E. Upper trachea
It is too big to have passed through the larynx. Think about the size of an endotracheal tube.

Answers: Extended Matching

7.13.1

A. Alcohol

Teenagers experimenting with alcohol can become intoxicated quickly. Drinking patterns in teenagers tend to be more extreme, with large amounts of alcohol consumed in very short periods. Alcohol drops the blood glucose level and can cause them to become comatose.

Cannabis would usually result in red eyes with dilated pupils. MDMA results in agitation but neither of these would provoke hypoglycaemia.

7.13.2

G. Paracetamol

This is likely to be a paracetamol overdose with delayed presentation, as her liver function has already been affected. This can be treated with N-acetylcysteine. Teenagers can deny taking anything, especially if asked with their parents present.

7.13.3

I. Salicylates (aspirin)

This is likely to be salicylate poisoning. The first stage of toxicity is characterized by hyperventilation resulting from direct respiratory centre stimulation, leading to a respiratory alkalosis.

7.13.4

F. Iron.

Iron can turn your stools black. If the black stools were melaena you would expect additional symptoms or signs. The presence of iron tablets at home would be a crucial aspect to the history.

7.13.5

D. Digoxin.

Treatment is with activated charcoal if the child presents <1 hour after ingestion. The child should have ECG monitoring and serum digoxin concentration measured. To be sure that this wasn't a tricyclic overdose (or indeed a red herring altogether), a careful and quick check of Grandma's actual medication, via her GP if necessary, can be very helpful.

Child protection

Questions: Single Best Answer

8.1

Alfie is a 2-year-old boy who presents to the Emergency Department with a painful right leg. His grandmother reports that he had fallen down the stairs earlier that day. He has not been walking on his leg since then. She thought he had pulled a muscle. On returning home, his parents brought him to the hospital. He has no other injuries and his development is normal for his age.

The X-ray is shown in Fig. 8.1.

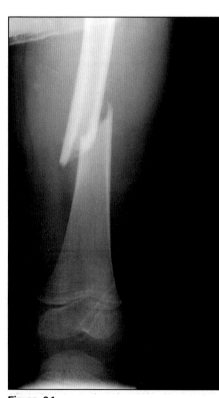

Figure 8.1

What is the most likely cause of this finding?

Select on answer only.

A. Accidental Injury
B. Non-accidental injury
C. Osteogenesis imperfecta (brittle bone disease)
D. Osteosarcoma
E. Vitamin D deficiency

8.2

You are a junior doctor working on the paediatric ward. You are asked to take some bloods from Chloe, an 11-year-old girl. Her parents do not wish to be present. When rolling up her sleeve to look for a suitable place for venepuncture you note numerous bruises from strap marks to her upper arm. You ask her how she got the bruising. She replies that her uncle did it as she had been naughty. She does not want you to tell her parents.

What should you do with the information?

Select on answer only.

A. Document what was said in the medical notes including sketches and inform the consultant on call
B. Document what was said in the notes including sketches and where possible photographs
C. Ignore it; she was being disciplined for misbehaviour and she has expressed her desire that no-one else is informed
D. Inform the health visitor and request a home assessment
E. Inform her mother what she said and suggest she asks the uncle about it

8.3

Pauline is a 6-year-old girl. Her teacher is concerned, as she has been rubbing herself 'down below' in the classroom and touching other girls. She later discloses to her teacher that her stepfather has hurt her with his 'willy'. She is seen by the consultant paediatrician who notices some vulval soreness and so takes a swab which reveals gonococcus. She also notices that there is some bruising to the thighs. She plots her weight and finds it to be just above the 99th centile. She has no other medical problems.

Which of the following findings is the most suggestive of sexual abuse?

Select one answer only.

A. Bruising to the thighs
B. Disclosure of event to teacher
C. Gonococcus on swab
D. Sexualised behaviour
E. Vulval soreness

8.4

Chelsea is a 2-year-old girl who presented 6 months ago with a fractured femur which was felt to be accidental. She presents to the Emergency Department having slipped in the bath whilst briefly being left alone. On examination there is swelling and bruising over Chelsea's anterior right chest wall. She has some older bruises on her right thigh. She has no other medical problems and is not on any medication. The chest X-ray (Fig. 8.2) reveals rib fractures.

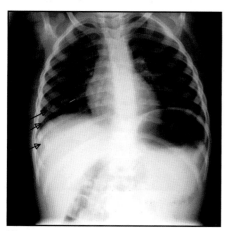

Figure 8.2

What is the most appropriate next step in management?

Select one answer only.

A. Check vitamin D status
B. Discharge home with follow up by GP the next day
C. Ensure a child protection medical takes place
D. Genetic counselling
E. Health visitor home assessment

Questions: Extended Matching

8.5
The following (A–I) is a list of possible diagnoses. For each of the children described in the following scenarios pick the most likely diagnosis. Each answer may be used once, more than once, or not at all.

A. Accidental injury
B. Acute allergic reaction
C. Acute lymphoblastic leukaemia
D. Immune thrombocytopenic purpura (ITP)
E. Meningococcal septicaemia
F. Non-accidental injury
G. Poisoning
H. Scald
I. Staphylococcal scalded skin infection

8.5.1
Ilsa is an 18-month-old child. Her mother has brought her to the Emergency Department with the marks on her left arm shown in Fig. 8.3. She had been at her father's house with her siblings all weekend and returned to her mother's care on Sunday night. Her mother asked her father what had happened and he had said he thought that she knocked herself on the coffee table.

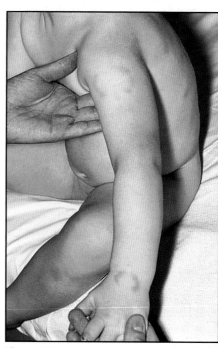

Figure 8.3

8.5.2
Mona a 3-month-old child presents to the Emergency Department as her parents are worried by the appearance of the right lower leg. On examination she has a temperature of 38.5°C and her leg is as shown in Fig. 8.4. Her mother reports that she had an infection around her mouth which she caught at nursery.

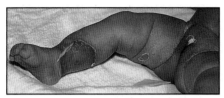

Figure 8.4

8.5.3
Aisha, a 6-year-old girl, is brought by her mother to the paediatric emergency clinic because of bruises. The family say that she had a viral upper respiratory tract infection (URTI) the previous week for which she saw her general practitioner. The URTI had completely resolved. She was well when she went to spend a long weekend with relatives but returned with multiple bruises. On examination she is well in herself and is afebrile. There is no hepatosplenomegaly. The appearance of her legs is shown in Fig. 8.5, and there is a bruise around her eye and a few scattered petechiae.

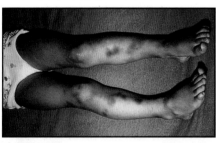

Figure 8.5

8.5.4
Denisa is a 14-year-old girl who presents to the Accident and Emergency department with fever and lethargy. On examination she is unwell and has a rash over all her body which is shown in Fig. 8.6. This rash does not disappear on applying pressure.

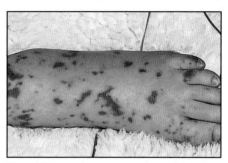

Figure 8.6

8.5.5
Lucy is a 22-month-old girl. She is brought to the Emergency Department by her mother. She was playing in the kitchen when her mother says she pulled a kettle of boiling water over her legs. The remainder of her examination is normal. She is in pain. Her legs are shown in Fig. 8.7. She has no other medical problems and is not on any medications.

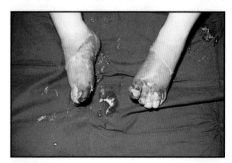

Figure 8.7

Answers: Single Best Answer

8.1

A. Accidental injury ⊘
Correct. There is an oblique midshaft fracture of the femur. The most common cause is an accident, though non-accidental injury always has to be borne in mind.

B. Non-accidental injury
The most common cause is an accident, though non-accidental injury always has to be borne in mind.

C. Osteogenesis imperfecta (brittle bone disease)
There is no evidence on the X-ray of generalised bone disease.

E. Osteosarcoma
Although bone tumours may predispose to fractures there is no evidence of a bone tumour on the X-ray.

D. Vitamin D deficiency
There is no evidence on the X-ray of rickets.

8.2

A. Document what was said in the medical notes including sketches and inform the Consultant on call. ⊘
Correct. This is a safeguarding issue, as the girl has alleged physical abuse and this needs to be taken seriously. Other agencies, e.g. social services need to be contacted to identify any concerns, and the patient needs a full medical examination by a paediatrician trained in child protection. Photographs will be helpful but consent must be obtained for these first. It is vital that the consultant on call knows what is happening and is involved.

B. Document what was said in the notes including sketches and where possible photographs
This is helpful but vital time may be lost in ensuring that all injuries are identified.
There may be more occult problems and it is better to get consultant involvement from the outset.

C. Ignore it; she was being disciplined for misbehaviour and she has expressed her desire that no-one else is informed
You are not bound by the duty of confidentiality in this instance. It is important to know the exceptions to this. See: http://www.gmc-uk.org/guidance/ethical_guidance/confidentiality.asp for more details and case discussions.

D. Inform the health visitor and request a home assessment
The first action is to record the findings carefully before a strategy meeting is arranged.

E. Inform her mother what she said and suggest she asks the uncle about it
The parents will need to be informed and consent should be sought for a full child protection medical.

8.3

A. Bruising to the thighs
Bruising over the thighs is common in active children but it is more concerning if it is found in the inner thigh as this area is anatomically 'protected' and not often bruised accidentally.

B. Disclosure of event to teacher
The disclosure is very useful and a police investigation would need to be undertaken.

C. Gonococcus on swab ⊘
Correct. All of these answers could suggest sexual abuse but only the gonococcus on the swab confirms it. It will not however inform you of whom the perpetrator is.

D. Sexualised behaviour
Sexualized behaviour may raise awareness of abuse as a potential problem but is not confirmatory of it.

E. Vulval soreness
Vulval soreness is common in young girls.

8.4

A. Check vitamin D status
Bruising over the chest wall is uncommon and rib fractures without a reasonable explanation (e.g. involvement in significant road traffic accident) are pathognomonic of abusive injury. Even if vitamin D is low, it would not explain these injuries.

B. Discharge home with follow up by GP the next day
Inappropriate under these circumstances.

C. Ensure a child protection medical takes place ⊘
Correct. Even if you do not see the fractures on this X-ray, there are some features in this history which are very concerning. The child is left unsupervised in the bath; she has had a previous femur fracture and has bruises on her thigh. A child protection medical review needs to be undertaken now by a consultant and a place of safety found for this child. This is usually in hospital but sometimes an alternative place of safety can be identified quickly.

D. Genetic counselling
Genetic counselling is not required.

E. Health visitor home assessment
A health visitor home assessment would be useful in this situation to gain more information but it would not be the most appropriate next step for this child.

Answers: Extended Matching

8.5.1
F. Non-accidental injury
This picture is consistent with a bite mark. There appear to be two bite marks. There is a smaller mark over the hand which is from a child, and it is not uncommon for toddlers to bite other children. However, the mark on the upper arm is consistent with a much older child or adult and as there is no adequate explanation, it is suggestive of a non-accidental injury. To be sure a forensic dentist may be helpful.

8.5.2
I. Staphylococcal scalded skin syndrome
This is staphylococcal scalded skin syndrome, caused by an exfoliative staphylococcal toxin which causes separation of the epidermal skin through the granular cell layers. This affects infants and young children. They develop fever and malaise, may have a purulent, crusting, localized infection around the eyes, nose, and mouth with subsequent widespread erythema and tenderness of the skin. Areas of epidermis separate on gentle pressure (Nikolsky's sign) leaving denuded areas of skin, as shown here, which subsequently dry and heal without scarring.

8.5.3
D. ITP (Immune thrombocytopenic purpura)
This is likely to be ITP. It classically follows a viral illness and here there is widespread purpura and bruising. A full blood count would reveal a low platelet count. If it were acute lymphoblastic leukaemia, she would be likely to be unwell and have other abnormal symptoms and signs, e.g. a febrile illness, splenomegaly.

8.5.4
E. Meningococcal septicaemia
This is meningococcal sepsis and immediate treatment with intravenous antibiotics is necessary. Her airway, breathing and circulation all need to be supported.

8.5.5
F. Non-accidental injury
This is a non-accidental injury. The image here shows what is known as 'glove and stocking' distribution of a burn on her feet. This type of scald indicates that the feet have been purposefully held in hot water. If a kettle had caused this there would not be such uniform demarcation and it is likely that there would be satellite lesions from splashes.

Genetics

Questions: Single Best Answer

9.1
Michael is a 6-year-old boy who is prone to bleeding. He has a problem with one of his clotting factors and his parents have been told that this is caused by a faulty gene. He is otherwise well and has no other medical problems. His parents have an appointment with the geneticist who takes a family history and draws a family tree, which is shown in Fig. 9.1.

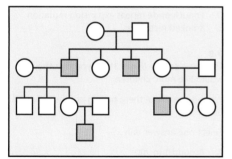

Figure 9.1

What is the most likely pattern of inheritance in this disorder?

Select one answer only.

A. Autosomal dominant
B. Autosomal recessive
C. Imprinting from uniparental disomy
D. Trinucleotide repeat expansion mutation
E. X-linked recessive

 Hint: Why are only squares affected?

9.2
The female marked with an arrow in Fig. 9.2 is planning on starting a family. If she were to give birth to a son, what would be the risk of him being affected by the disorder?

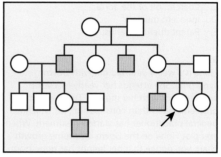

Figure 9.2

Select one answer only.

A. 1 in 1
B. 1 in 2
C. 1 in 3
D. 1 in 4
E. 1 in 5

9.3
Mr and Mrs Walsh attend the clinic with their new baby, Ophelia, who has Down syndrome. They are keen to have further children and want to know more about their future risk of having children with Down syndrome. What chromosomal abnormality is likely to have caused Ophelia to have Down syndrome?

Select one answer only.

A. Mosaicism
B. Nondisjunction
C. Point mutation
D. Translocation
E. Triplet repeat expansion

9.4
Mr and Mrs David are seen by the geneticists as their baby, Sarah, has Down syndrome. Her chromosomes are examined. Three copies of chromosome 21 are seen, one of which is attached to chromosome 14. How would you describe this abnormality?

Select one answer only.

A. Balanced Robertsonian translocation
B. Mosaicism
C. Nondisjunction
D. Triplet repeat expansion
E. Unbalanced Robertsonian translocation

9.5
Olive is a 10-day-old baby with Down syndrome. On examination, you hear a loud heart murmur. What is the most likely cause?

Select one answer only.

A. Aortic stenosis
B. Atrioventricular septal defect
C. Coarctation of the aorta
D. Innocent murmur
E. Patent ductus arteriosus

9.6
Fiona is a well 4-year-old girl with Down syndrome. She attends her yearly follow-up appointment with her mother. There are no real problems other than constipation, for which her general practitioner has started treatment. When you plot Fiona on the Down syndrome growth chart, you notice that her height has gone from the 75th centile to the 25th centile. Her weight, however, has gone from the 50th centile to the 75th centile.

Which of the following investigations would you perform?

Select one answer only.

A. Coeliac screen
B. Abdominal ultrasound
C. Full blood count
D. Thyroid function tests
E. Vitamin D levels

9.7
Mary is an infant with Down syndrome. Her antenatal scans had all been normal and an echocardiogram on the neonatal unit shortly after birth was normal. She attends the community clinic for the first time at 4 weeks of age. She is now thriving and feeding well. Her parents have many questions about what is going to happen in the future. In particular, they have been reading that she is still at an increased risk of certain diseases because she has Down syndrome.

Out of the following, which condition is Mary at increased risk of developing compared with the general population?

Select one answer only.

A. Congenital heart disease
B. Duodenal atresia

C. Ischaemic heart disease
D. Leukaemia
E. Pyloric stenosis

9.8
A Pakistani couple are referred for genetic counselling. They have lost two children who both died in the first 2 years of life. They have one healthy girl, who is 3 years of age. The faulty gene has been identified and other members of their family have been tested (Fig. 9.3).

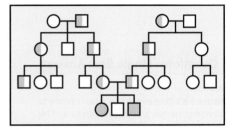

Figure 9.3

What is the pattern of inheritance in this disorder?

A. Autosomal dominant
B. Autosomal recessive
C. Imprinting from uniparental disomy
D. Trinucleotide repeat expansion mutation
E. X-linked recessive

9.9
The same couple (Fig. 9.3) tell you that they would like more children.

What is the risk of them having another affected baby?

Select one answer only.

A. Around 1 in 200
B. 1 in 2
C. 1 in 4
D. 2 in 3
E. 3 in 4

9.10
A Bangladeshi couple are referred for genetic counselling. Both parents are carriers of a faulty gene *PEX1*; possession of two abnormal copies of this gene leads to death in infancy. They have lost two children who both died in the first 2 years of life. They have one healthy daughter, who is 3 years of age. What is the risk that their daughter is a carrier?

A. None
B. 1 in 4
C. 1 in 2
D. 2 in 3
E. 100%

9.11

Gemma and Mark, who are both well, are planning to start a family. Gemma's older brother has cystic fibrosis. There is no history of cystic fibrosis in Mark's family. The family tree is shown in Fig. 9.4. What is the chance that they will have a child with cystic fibrosis? The carrier rate is 1 in 25 in their population.

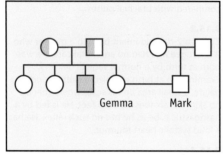

Figure 9.4

Select one answer only.

A. 1 in 6
B. 1 in 37.5
C. 1 in 100
D. 1 in 150
E. 1 in 2500

9.12

A mother comes to see the geneticist. She has two children, Robert and Elizabeth. They both suffer from a genetic disorder. The geneticist takes a history and draws the family tree (Fig. 9.5).

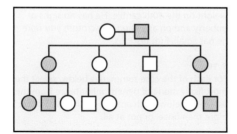

Figure 9.5

What is the likely pattern of inheritance in this disorder?

Select one answer only.

A. Autosomal dominant
B. Autosomal recessive
C. Imprinting from uniparental disomy
D. X-linked dominant
E. X-linked recessive

9.13

George has Klinefelter syndrome. What is his karyotype?

Select one answer only.

A. 46, XO
B. 46, XY
C. 45, XO
D. 45, XY
E. 47, XXY

9.14

Louise (Fig. 9.6) is a 14-year-old girl. She is attending the endocrinology clinic, as she is the shortest girl in her class and wants to know if there is treatment to make her taller. She is otherwise well and has no other medical complaints. She has always been the shortest girl in her class. Her clinical appearance is shown in the picture. Her height plots well below the 0.4th centile but her weight is on the 9th centile. Her chromosome karyotype is 46, XX.

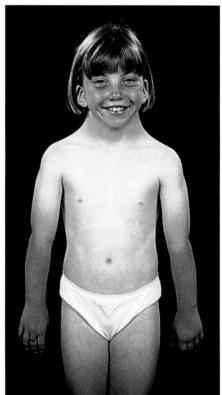

Figure 9.6

What is the most likely cause of her short stature.

Select one answer only.

A. Cushing syndrome
B. Down syndrome
C. Noonan syndrome
D. Turner syndrome
E. Normal variant (constitutional short stature)

Questions: Extended Matching

9.15
The following (A–N) is a list of genetic disorders. For each child described select the most likely genetic diagnosis from the list. Each answer may be used, more than once, or not at all.

A. Achondroplasia
B. Angelman syndrome
C. Cystic fibrosis
D. Down syndrome
E. Duchenne muscular dystrophy
F. Edward syndrome
G. Fragile X syndrome
H. Klinefelter syndrome
I. Neurofibromatosis
J. Noonan syndrome
K. Patau syndrome
L. Prader–Willi syndrome
M. Turner syndrome
N. Williams syndrome

9.15.1
Rachael is a 3-month-old girl who attends the Emergency Department because of rapid breathing. She is the 5th infant born to a 39-year-old mother. When you take her developmental history, you find she smiled at 7 weeks but is unable to hold her head unsupported. On examination, she is tachypnoeic, sweaty and hypotonic. Her clinical appearance can be seen in Fig. 9.7. You plot her weight and she is below the 0.4th centile.

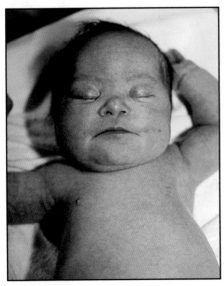

Figure 9.7

9.15.2
Amelia is a 14-year-old girl who has not started puberty. Her friends at school have all started their periods but she hasn't even started any breast development. She is an otherwise well girl with no other medical complaints. Her mother mentions she had puffy hands and feet as a baby. On examination you note that she is short (<0.4th centile for height) and has a systolic heart murmur and diminished femoral pulse pressure compared with brachial pulses.

9.15.3
Cyril is a 2-day-old infant born to a mother who is a refugee and had no antenatal care. He was born at term by a normal vaginal delivery. Examination at birth revealed a cleft lip and palate, a small area on his scalp where there is no skin and six toes on both feet. He is fed by a nasogastric tube as he has no suck reflex. He has a loud systolic heart murmur.

9.15.4
Rafael is a 6-year-old boy. He is referred to the paediatric outpatient department by the school nurse. His class teacher reports that he finds most learning activities very difficult. His behaviour is difficult to manage in class. On examination you note that he has a large head which plots on the 99th centile. His height and weight are on the 25th centile. He has a long face and large ears. The remainder of examination is normal.

9.15.5
Roger is a 12-year-old boy. He is referred to the paediatric outpatient department because he has developed breasts. His class teacher reports that his behaviour is difficult to manage in class. On examination you note that he is very tall and slim, with his height on the 99th centile and his weight on the 40th centile. He has no signs of puberty and on assessing his scrotum you note he has small, firm testicles.

9.16
For each of the case summaries below, select the most likely mode of genetic inheritance from the list (A–G) below. Each answer can be used once, more than once, or not at all.

A. Autosomal dominant disorder
B. Autosomal recessive disorder
C. Imprinting from uniparental disomy
D. Microdeletion
E. Polygenic
F. X-linked dominant
G. X-linked recessive

9.16.1
Jack is a 3-year-old boy whose father has a genetic disorder associated with short stature. Jack is also very short, has bowed legs and a very prominent forehead. His head is

disproportionately large compared with his body size.

9.16.2
Mercy is a 7-month-old, Black-African girl who presents to the Emergency Department with fever and severe pain in her digits. She has a past medical history of being chronically tired. On examination you note that she has pale conjunctiva and mild hepatomegaly. She is febrile and appears to have an upper respiratory tract infection. Her fingers are swollen.

9.16.3
Bruce is a 12-year-old boy who is referred by the ophthalmology team. He presented with blurred vision. Ophthalmological examination revealed a dislocated lens. He is very disappointed, as he had been doing very well in his basketball team.

He is also doing well academically at school. On examination you note he is very tall. He has a high arched palate, stretch marks on his skin and lax joints. His height is well above the 99th centile and he has long arms, legs, and fingers. His mother is also tall (178 cm) but reports that she is healthy.

9.16.4
A child is suspected of having Prader-Willi syndrome. This is confirmed on genetic analysis but there is no deletion of genetic material.

9.16.5
Gregor, aged 6 weeks, is vomiting his feeds. His vomit is 'like a fountain', and immediately afterwards he is hungry again. When examined after a vomit, a mass could be felt in the right upper quadrant of his abdomen.

Answers: Single Best Answer

9.1
A. Autosomal dominant
It could only be autosomal dominant if there was incomplete and variable penetrance of this condition.

B. Autosomal recessive
Whilst it is theoretically possible to see a pattern like this in autosomal recessive conditions it would be highly unlikely. Both great grandparents would have to be carriers and two 'new' partners would also have to be carriers. Unlikely unless there is significant consanguinity.

C. Imprinting from uniparental disomy
Following meiosis, imprinting proceeds in a 'parent of origin' specific manner. In general this 'resets' the genetic information correctly and therefore uniparental disomy is not heritable.

D. Trinucleotide repeat expansion mutation
This would result in genetic anticipation where the disease would be more severe or be evident sooner in subsequent generations.

E. X-linked recessive ⊘
Correct. Only males are affected and females can be carriers. Very rarely female carriers can show mild signs and symptoms. An example of such a genetic disorder is haemophilia A.

9.2
A. 1 in 1
This would be close to the risk if she had a mitochondrial disorder.

B. 1 in 2
This would be the risk if she was a known carrier.

C. 1 in 3
Risks can deviate from expected ratios if diseases are fatal in utero. But this is not the case.

D. 1 in 4 ⊘
Correct. There are two questions to answer:
(1) What is the risk that this person has the faulty gene and then (2) what is the risk of passing it on?
This is an X-linked recessive disorder. As her brother is affected, her mother is a carrier. The female in question therefore has a 50% chance of also being a carrier. If she were to have a son there would be a further 50% chance of passing this condition on. Therefore there is a total 25% risk (1 in 4) of her son being affected.

E. 1 in 5
It is very hard to get a situation where the risk of recurrence is 1 in 5.

9.3
A. Mosaicism
This accounts for about 1% of cases

B. Nondisjunction ⊘
Correct. Meiotic nondisjunction accounts for 94% of cases of Down syndrome. Most cases are a result of an error at meiosis.

C. Point mutation
No, Down syndrome is a trisomy. There is an extra copy of an entire chromosome (21).

D. Translocation
This accounts for 5% of cases. It must be unbalanced to result in the clinical syndrome.

E. Triplet repeat expansion
No, Down syndrome is a trisomy. There is an extra copy of an entire chromosome (21).

9.4
A. Balanced Robertsonian translocation
Balanced translocations do not result in clinical features but increase the risk of having a child with the condition.

B. Mosaicism
In mosaicism some of the cells are normal and some have trisomy 21.

C. Nondisjunction
This would be more common and simply result in three copies of chromosome 21.

D. Triplet repeat expansion
This would result in an alteration in the DNA sequence, often in a noncoding region (intron).

E. Unbalanced Robertsonian translocation ⊘
Correct. This is important because there is an increased risk of recurrence as one of the parents is likely to have a balanced translocation whereby one of their copies of chromosome 21 is attached to chromosome 14.

9.5
A. Aortic stenosis
It does occur in children with Down syndrome but it is much less common than atrioventricular septal defect and ventricular septal defect.

B. Atrioventricular septal defect ⊘
Correct. This is the most common congenital cardiac anomaly in children with Down syndrome. 40% of children with Down syndrome have a congenital heart defect and therefore, all children with Down syndrome should have an echocardiogram in the neonatal period.

C. Coarctation of the aorta
It does occur in children with Down syndrome but it is much less common than atrioventricular septal defect and ventricular septal defect.

D. Innocent murmur
It would be unusual for an innocent murmur to be loud. They are usually 'soft, short, systolic, localized in site, and there are no signs or symptoms'.

E. Patent ductus arteriosus
Common in preterm babies but not the typical abnormality seen in a child with Down syndrome.

9.6
A. Coeliac antibodies
Whilst children with Down syndrome are at increased risk of coeliac disease this is usually associated with faltering growth.

B. Abdominal ultrasound
Unhelpful in this situation.

C. Full blood count
Children with Down syndrome are at increased risk of leukaemia – but this is not the correct clinical history.

D. Thyroid function tests ⊘
Correct. Children with Down syndrome are at an increased risk of hypothyroidism. Growth failure and constipation are symptoms of hypothyroidism.

E. Vitamin D levels
Severe vitamin D deficiency might cause a reduction in height but not an increase in weight and is not more common in children with Down syndrome.

9.7
A. Congenital heart disease
Her echocardiogram is normal though. Therefore her risk is not increased.

B. Duodenal atresia
This would have presented soon after birth.

C. Ischaemic heart disease
There is no increased risk of this ischaemic heart disease in children with Down syndrome.

D. Leukaemia ⊘
Correct. Children with Down syndrome are at increased risk of leukaemia.

E. Pyloric stenosis
No increased risk.

9.8
A. Autosomal dominant
There are carriers shown.

B. Autosomal recessive ⊘
Correct. Autosomal recessive conditions are more commonly seen in families with consanguinity.

C. Imprinting from uniparental disomy
Following meiosis, imprinting proceeds in a 'parent of origin' specific manner. In general this 'resets' the genetic information correctly and therefore uniparental disomy is not heritable.

D. Trinucleotide repeat expansion mutation
The inheritance of trinucleotide repeat expansion disorders is usually autosomal dominant. The key feature would be one of 'genetic anticipation': it would be clinically more severe in each generation.

E. X-linked recessive
There are male carriers evident in the family tree.

9.9
A. Around 1 in 200
This is the recurrence risk of Down syndrome for a mother under 35 years of age if the underlying cause was nondisjunction.

B. 1 in 2
This is the recurrence risk of autosomal dominant conditions when one parent is affected or X-linked recessive conditions where mother is a carrier.

C. 1 in 4 ⊘
Correct. This is an autosomal recessive condition. If both parents are carriers for an autosomal recessive condition then there is a 1 in 4 chance of a child being affected.

D. 2 in 3
This is the recurrence risk of an autosomal dominant condition when homozygosity is associated with fetal death and both parents carry the gene.

E. 3 in 4
This is the recurrence risk of an autosomal dominant condition when homozygosity results in liveborn children and both parents have the condition.

9.10
A. None
Whilst it is clear that she does not possess two copies of the faulty gene (she is healthy), she may be a carrier.

B. 1 in 4
There is a 1 in 4 chance of a future pregnancy resulting in an affected child, but this is not the clinical scenario.

C. 1 in 2
There is a 1 in 2 chance that a pregnancy will result in a child being a carrier. However, this is a subtly different question, as one possibility does not exist as this child is definitely not affected.

D. 2 in 3 ⊘
Correct. As she does not have the condition, there are three possible outcomes, one (1 in 3) is that she is not a carrier, the other two (2 in 3) are that she is a carrier.

E. 100%
This is incorrect as there is a possibility that parents passed on their 'good' copies of gene *PEX1*. (This is the gene responsible for one form of Zellweger syndrome, a rare but fatal condition resulting in defective peroxisomes).

9.11

A. 1 in 6
This would be the risk if Mark was known to be a carrier but Gemma's status was unknown. A more complicated pedigree where Mark already has an affected child by another partner could give this risk.

B. 1 in 37.5
This is roughly the risk that both parents are carriers. As Gemma does not have the condition there are three possible outcomes, one (33%) is that she is not a carrier, the other two (66%) are that she is a carrier, i.e. $2/3 \times 1/25 = 1$ in 37.5.

C. 1 in 100
This is a tempting option but incorrect. If Gemma was known to be a carrier and she found a partner from the general population, this would be the chance that a pregnancy would result in an affected child, i.e. $1/25 \times 1/4 = 1/100$.

D. 1 in 150 ⊘
Correct. As Gemma does not have the condition there are three possible outcomes, one (1 in 3) is that she is not a carrier, the other two (2 in 3) are that she is a carrier. The risk of Mark being an unaffected carrier is the population frequency of heterozygosity. The risk of two carriers having an affected child is 1 in 4 per pregnancy. Therefore the risk is roughly $2/3 \times 1/25 \times 1/4$. This could be refined slightly if Gemma's status is known, but this might not influence the couples decision about screening. Checking whether Mark is a carrier has a bigger influence on the risk.

E. 1 in 2500
This is incorrect but is the risk for Caucasian couples having a child with cystic fibrosis in the UK.

9.12

A. Autosomal dominant ⊘
Correct. This is the most common mode of Mendelian inheritance. An affected individual carries the abnormal gene in the heterozygous state. Offspring have a 50% chance of inheriting the abnormal gene.

B. Autosomal recessive
Providing that new partners came from outside this family, the chance that this pattern is autosomal recessive is extremely low.

C. Imprinting from uniparental disomy
Following meiosis, imprinting proceeds in a 'parent of origin' specific manner. In general this 'resets' the genetic information correctly and therefore uniparental disomy is not heritable.

D. X-linked dominant
In X-linked dominant inheritance all the daughters of an affected male have the condition as he must pass on a copy of the gene to any daughter.

E. X-linked recessive
Males and females are equally affected in this family's pedigree therefore, it cannot be X-linked recessive.

9.13

A. 46, XO
An interesting karyotype. This could only occur if you had an extra autosome and a missing sex chromosome.

B. 46, XY
Normal male karyotype.

C. 45, XO
Turner syndrome.

D. 45, XY
There is a missing autosome. This would not be survivable.

E. 47, XXY ⊘
Correct. This is Klinefelter syndrome.

9.14

A. Cushing syndrome
In Cushing syndrome there is growth failure but you would also expect other clinical features as listed in Box 9.1.

Box 9.1 Clinical features of Cushing syndrome

- Growth failure/short stature
- Face and trunk obesity
- Red cheeks
- Hirsutism
- Striae
- Hypertension
- Bruising
- Carbohydrate intolerance
- Muscle wasting and weakness
- Osteopenia
- Psychological problems.

B. Down syndrome
Children with Down syndrome are small but have different clinical features. See Box 9.2.

C. Noonan syndrome ⊘
Correct. She has a round face with short, webbed neck, and short stature since infancy, characteristic of Noonan syndrome. There is some overlap with the phenotype of Turner syndrome, but her karyotype is normal.

D. Turner syndrome
The normal karyotype excludes Turner syndrome.

Box 9.2 Characteristic clinical manifestations of Down syndrome

Typical craniofacial appearance

- Round face and flat nasal bridge
- Upslanted palpebral fissures
- Epicanthic folds (a fold of skin running across the inner edge of the palpebral fissure)
- Brushfield spots in iris (pigmented spots)
- Small mouth and protruding tongue
- Small ears
- Flat occiput and third fontanelle

Other anomalies

- Short neck
- Single palmar creases, incurved and short fifth finger and wide 'sandal' gap between first and second toes
- Hypotonia
- Congenital heart defects (in 40%)
- Duodenal atresia
- Hirschsprung disease (<1%)

Later medical problems

- Delayed motor milestones
- Learning difficulties – severity is variable, usually mild to moderate but may be severe
- Short stature
- Increased susceptibility to infections
- Hearing impairment from secretory otitis media (75%)
- Visual impairment from cataracts (15%), squints, myopia (50%)
- Increased risk of leukaemia and solid tumours (<1%)
- Acquired hip dislocation and atlanto-axial instability
- Obstructive sleep apnoea (50–75%)
- Increased risk of hypothyroidism (15%) and coeliac disease
- Epilepsy
- Early onset Alzheimer disease.

E. Normal variant (constitutional short stature)
Not with the clinical features shown.

Answers: Extended Matching

9.15.1
D. Down syndrome
The picture shows the facial features of Down syndrome – round face with a flat nose, upslanted palpebral fissures and epicanthic folds (a fold of skin running across the inner edge of the palpebral fissure). Other features are her hypotonia. Her mother's older age increases her risk of having a child with Down syndrome. The tachypnoea, sweatiness and poor weight gain could reflect heart failure from congenital heart disease. Plotting her weight on a Down syndrome chart would be more appropriate.

9.15.2
M. Turner syndrome
Features include delayed puberty, primary amenorrhoea, short stature, coarctation of the aorta and lymphoedema as a neonate. Noonan syndrome shares many of these features.

9.15.3
K. Patau syndrome (trisomy 13)
Cyril has a cleft lip and palate, a scalp defect, polydactyly, and a heart defect. These are all features of Patau syndrome.

9.15.4
G. Fragile X syndrome
Fragile X is one of the most common causes of learning difficulties in boys. Characteristic features are a long face with large everted ears.

The mandible is often prominent, with a broad forehead. They have macro-orchidism post-puberty. See Box 9.3 and Fig. 9.8.

Box 9.3 Clinical findings in males with fragile X syndrome

- Moderate–severe learning difficulty (IQ 20–80, mean 50)
- Macrocephaly
- Macro-orchidism – postpubertal
- Characteristic facies – long face, large everted ears, prominent mandible, and broad forehead, most evident in affected adults
- Other features – mitral valve prolapse, joint laxity, scoliosis, autism, hyperactivity.

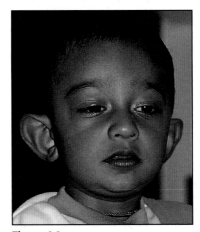

Figure 9.8

9.15.5
H. Klinefelter syndrome

9.16.1
A. Autosomal dominant disorder
Jack and his father have the same condition. Jack has achondroplasia.

9.16.2
B. Autosomal recessive disorder
Mercy has sickle cell disease. Carrier status is protective against malaria and has resulted in a high incidence of this condition in populations who originate from endemic areas as heterozygote status confers a survival benefit.

9.16.3
A. Autosomal dominant disorder
Bruce has Marfan syndrome. The causes of tall stature are described in Table 9.1. Whilst the description alone could suggest an X-linked dominant inheritance, conditions that are inherited in this manner are rare.

Table 9.1 Causes of excessive growth or tall stature

Familial	Most common cause
Obesity	Puberty is advanced, so final height centile is less than in childhood
Secondary	Hyperthyroidism Excess sex steroids – precocious puberty from whatever cause Excess adrenal androgen steroids – congenital adrenal hyperplasia True gigantism (excess growth hormone secretion)

Syndromes	Long-legged tall stature
	    Marfan syndrome
	    Homocystinuria
	    Klinefelter syndrome (47, XXY karyotype)
	Sotos syndrome – associated with large head, characteristic facial features and learning difficulties

9.16.4
C. Imprinting from uniparental disomy
Uniparental disomy accounts for 10% of Prader–Willi syndrome. A child who inherits two maternal copies of chromosome 15 will have Prader-Willi syndrome from imprinting. See Fig. 9.9.

Imprinting from a uniparental disomy

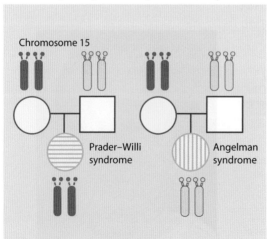

Chromosome 15

Prader–Willi syndrome

Angelman syndrome

Figure 9.9

Answer 9.16.5
E. Polygenic

Gregor has pyloric stenosis. This is a classic polygenic disorder. It is more common in boys than girls and this unequal sex incidence leads to the Carter phenomenon, where an affected female is more likely to pass the condition on to her children than an affected male. This is because there is a sex specific threshold for expression of pyloric stenosis that is lower in males. Affected females are more likely to pass it on.

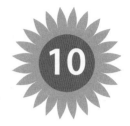

Perinatal medicine

Questions: Single Best Answer

10.1

A mother has just found out she is pregnant and asks for advice about how to look after her health and nutrition during pregnancy. She smokes 15 cigarettes a day. You recommend she gives up smoking.

If she continues to smoke despite your advice the baby is at increased risk of which of the following health problems?

Select one answer only.

A. Growth restriction
B. Dysmorphic syndromes
C. Neural tube defects
D. Shoulder dystocia
E. Vitamin D deficiency

10.2

A mother has her routine 20-week antenatal scan. The sonographer finds the fetal abdominal and head circumference measurements are normal, but is concerned that there is an abnormally small amount of amniotic fluid (oligohydramnios).

What is the most likely cause for this.

Select one answer only.

A. Duodenal atresia
B. Gastroschisis
C. Maternal diabetes
D. Poorly functioning fetal kidneys
E. Severe intrauterine growth restriction

10.3

A midwife is concerned that a mother who is at 32 weeks' gestation has a symphysis–fundal height smaller than expected. An ultrasound confirms intrauterine growth restriction.

Which feature would be of most concern to the sonographer?

Select one answer only.

A. Accelerations of fetal heart rate
B. Active fetal movements

C. Breech presentation
D. Fetal breathing movements seen
E. Reverse end-diastolic flow in the umbilical artery

10.4

A mother has just found out she is pregnant with twins. Her antenatal scan reveals dichorionic, diamniotic twins.

Which condition carries the biggest increased risk in her twin pregnancy?

Select one answer only.

A. Congenital abnormalities
B. Gestational diabetes
C. Macrosomia
D. Post-term gestation
E. Twin-to-twin transfusion

10.5

You perform a routine newborn examination on a baby who is 20 hours old.

Which one of the following features requires further immediate assessment?

Select one answer only.

A. Acrocyanosis (cyanosis of the hands and feet)
B. A heart murmur
C. An undescended testis
D. Breast enlargement
E. Subconjunctival haemorrhages

10.6

A black mother is found to have glycosuria at her midwife appointment at 32 weeks' gestation. Her glucose tolerance test and fasting glucose is abnormal. She is given dietary advice to control her blood glucose.

What problem is her newborn baby at most increased risk of?

Select one answer only.

A. Anaemia
B. Hyperglycaemia
C. Respiratory distress syndrome

D. Neonatal bacterial infection
E. Neonatal type 1 diabetes mellitus

10.7
Jonathan, a newborn baby, is noted to have hepatosplenomegaly and a petechial rash. His red eye reflex is normal and there is no heart murmur. He fails his newborn screening hearing test. His mother is from the UK and her antenatal screening bloods were all normal.

What is the most likely congenital infection that has caused these symptoms?

Select one answer only.

A. Cytomegalovirus
B. Rubella
C. Syphilis
D. Toxoplasmosis
E. Varicella zoster

10.8
A male infant is born at term. At 1 minute of age he is breathing regularly and has a heart rate of 140 beats/min. He is grimacing but has not yet cried. He is pink centrally but still blue around his extremities and his tone is reduced although he has good limb flexion but is not actively moving his limbs.

What is his Apgar score at one minute?

Select one answer only.

A. 10
B. 9
C. 8
D. 7
E. 6

👆 **Hint: The measurement of Apgar score is shown in Chapter 10. Perinatal medicine in Illustrated Textbook of Paediatrics.**

10.9
A mother is known to have pre-eclampsia and her fetus has shown signs of intrauterine growth restriction on antenatal scans. He is delivered at 37 weeks and weighs 2.2 kg. He is admitted to the Special Care Baby Unit because of his size. He appears well and has had a breast feed.

What is he most at risk of?

Select one answer only.

A. Anaemia
B. Congenital cardiac abnormality
C. Group B streptococcus infection
D. Hypoglycaemia
E. Hypercalcaemia

10.10
In the UK all newborn babies have a heel-prick blood sample taken at 5–7 days of age for biochemical screening.

Which of the following is not tested for in the UK?

Select one answer only.

A. Cystic fibrosis
B. Duchenne muscular dystrophy
C. Hypothyroidism
D. Phenylketonuria
E. Sickle cell disease

10.11
Sam, a two-day-old infant, weighs 3.6 kg at birth. He was born by vaginal delivery with Apgar scores of 7 at 1 minute and 10 at 5 minutes. On day 2 he is reported to be jittery, crying inconsolably and feeding poorly. He sneezes and yawns, and is thought to have some abnormal movements, possibly seizures. No dysmorphic features are present and he is not jaundiced.

What is the most likely explanation for his problems?

Select one answer only.

A. Congenital rubella syndrome
B. Hypoxic-ischaemic encephalopathy
C. Fetal alcohol syndrome
D. Kernicterus
E. Maternal opiate use

10.12
Mohammed is 24 hours old. His mother develops chicken pox (varicella) 1 day after his delivery.

From the following list of options what is the best advice you could give?

Select one answer only.

A. Breastfeeding is contraindicated
B. Neonatal infection is unlikely due to transplacentally acquired antibodies
C. Reassure and discharge home asking mother to return if the baby develops symptoms.
D. The infant's varicella antibody status should be checked
E. There is a significant risk of serious neonatal infection

Questions: Extended Matching

10.13
From the following list (A–K) pick the diagnosis that fits best with the attached clinical description and picture. Each option may be used once, more than once, or not at all.

A. Bruising
B. Capillary haemangioma (stork bites)
C. Erythema toxicum (neonatal urticarial)
D. Group B streptococcal infection
E. Milia
F. Mongolian blue spots
G. Neonatal varicella zoster
H. Peripheral cyanosis
I. Port wine stain (naevus flammeus)
J. Strawberry naevus (cavernous haemangioma)
K. Traumatic cyanosis

10.13.1

George, a 2-day-old baby boy, is reviewed by the paediatric doctor at the request of the midwife. He was born by forceps delivery and has been feeding well. There were no risk factors for sepsis and mother was well during her pregnancy. When examined, he appears very well but has the rash shown in Fig. 10.1. His mother reports the rash keeps moving around his body.

 Hint: The baby looks well.

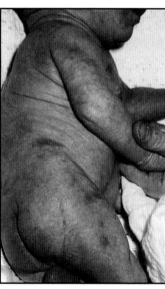

Figure 10.1

10.13.2

Anna, a month-old infant, is reviewed by the general practitioner. She was born by normal vaginal delivery, and was well during and after delivery. Her mother is worried about the mark on her face (Fig. 10.2). It has not changed in appearance since birth.

10.13.3

Oliver, a 4-day-old infant, is having a routine newborn check by the junior paediatric doctor.

The doctor notices some small white spots on Oliver's nose and cheeks (Fig. 10.3). Oliver was born by normal vaginal delivery and is currently feeding well.

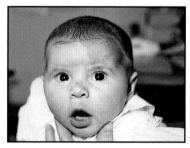

Figure 10.2

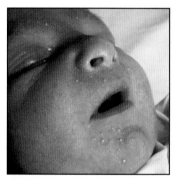

Figure 10.3

10.13.4

Jessica, a 2-month-old infant, presents to her family doctor with a mass on her forehead as shown in Fig. 10.4. It was not present at birth, and has been gradually increasing in size since it was first noticed when Jessica was about 3 weeks old. Jessica is well. The only past medical history of note is an uncomplicated premature delivery at 33 weeks gestation.

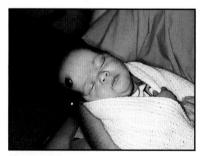

Figure 10.4

 Hint: It is raised and her mother is not too worried as her older brother had a similar lesion that resolved between 18 and 24 months.

10.13.5

Adam, a 3-day-old black infant, has his routine newborn check. The paediatric doctor notices blue and black macules on his back and buttocks (Fig. 10.5). Adam was born by normal vaginal delivery and has been feeding well since birth.

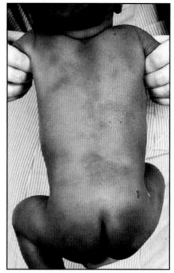

Figure 10.5

Answers: Single Best Answer

10.1
A. Being growth restricted ✓
Correct. Smoking reduces birthweight and is associated with increased risk of stillbirths and miscarriages. It also is known to adversely affect fetal lung growth.

B. Dysmorphic syndromes
Alcohol ingestion in pregnancy is associated with increased risk of fetal alcohol syndrome.

C. Neural tube defects
Folic acid should be taken by mothers prior to conception and in the first trimester to reduce the risk of neural tube defects.

D. Shoulder dystocia
Shoulder dystocia is associated with infants who are large for gestational age and is more common in mothers with gestational diabetes or poorly controlled diabetes.

E. Vitamin D deficiency
Smoking does not increase the risk of vitamin D deficiency.

10.2
A. Duodenal atresia
Duodenal atresia may be associated with polyhydramnios (excess amniotic fluid).

B. Gastroschisis
Gastroschisis should not affect the volume of amniotic fluid.

C. Maternal diabetes
Maternal diabetes may be associated with polyhydramnios (excess amniotic fluid).

D. Poorly functioning fetal kidneys ✓
Correct. Oligohydramnios, when there is reduced or lack of amniotic fluid, may be associated with decreased fetal urine output because of abnormal kidneys. Early scans will miss this problem as the fetal skin is not keratinised and amniotic fluid volume is proportional to fetal size. By 20 weeks it is dependent upon fetal urine production and that the membranes are intact.

E. Severe intrauterine growth restriction
Oligohydramnios may be associated with severe intrauterine growth restriction, but the sonographer has identified a normal head and abdominal circumference.

10.3
A. Accelerations of fetal heart rate
Accelerations of the fetal heart rate are a normal finding.

B. Active fetal movements
Active fetal movements are a normal sign. Reduced fetal movements would suggest fetal compromise.

C. Breech presentation
It is common for the baby to not have fully engaged at this stage of pregnancy.

D. Fetal breathing movements seen
Fetal breathing movements are a normal sign.

E. Reverse end-diastolic flow in the umbilical artery ✓
Correct. Absent or reversed flow velocity during diastole carries an increased risk of morbidity from hypoxic damage to the gut or brain, and of intrauterine death.

10.4
A. Congenital abnormalities ✓
Correct. There is a higher rate of congenital abnormalities in twin pregnancies. These occur twice as frequently as in a singleton (but the risk is increased four-fold in monochorionic twins).

B. Gestational diabetes
Multiple births do not significantly increase the mother's risk of gestational diabetes.

C. Macrosomia
Multiple births are at risk of intrauterine growth restriction rather than macrosomia.

D. Post-term gestation
Multiple births are at risk of preterm rather than post-term births. The median gestation for twins is 37 weeks, 34 weeks for triplets and 32 weeks for quadruplets.

E. Twin-to-twin transfusion
Twin–twin transfusion syndrome is found in monochorionic twins (with a shared placenta). She has dichorionic, diamniotic twins, and therefore they are not at risk of this as they have two separate placentas.

10.5
A. Acrocyanosis (cyanosis of the hands and feet)
This is common on the first day and resolves spontaneously.

B. A heart murmur ✓
Correct. Although many heart murmurs heard at the first day of life are innocent and will disappear, some are from congenital heart disease. Further clinical assessment is required to determine if the murmur is innocent or significant.

C. An undescended testis
Urgent surgical opinion for an undescended testis is not required as many descend spontaneously in the first few weeks of life, and surgical repair is therefore delayed. The testis should be rechecked at a few weeks of age.

D. Breast enlargement
Breast enlargement can occur in either sex and a small amount of milk may be discharged. This resolves spontaneously and does not require investigation.

E. Subconjunctival haemorrhages
These occur commonly during delivery and reassurance should be given.

10.6
A. Anaemia
These newborn infants are at increased risk of polycythaemia (venous haematocrit >0.65) rather than anaemia.

B. Hyperglycaemia
Transient hypoglycaemia is common during the first day of life in these infants due to fetal hyperinsulinism, which is in response to the high levels of maternal glucose crossing the placenta.

C. Respiratory distress syndrome ⊘
Correct. This mother has gestational diabetes which places the infant at increased risk of respiratory distress syndrome as lung maturation is delayed.

D. Neonatal bacterial infection
Infants of diabetic mothers are not at particular risk of neonatal infection.

E. Neonatal type 1 diabetes mellitus
There is no increased risk of neonatal type 1 diabetes mellitus in babies born to mothers with gestational diabetes.

10.7
A. Cytomegalovirus ⊘
Correct. This is the most common congenital infection in the UK. Most babies born to mothers with cytomegalovirus infection during pregnancy are normal at birth, but 5% have clinical features such as hepatosplenomegaly and petechiae and sensorineural hearing loss. Most of these babies will go on to have neurodevelopmental disabilities. 5% who appear normal at birth develop sensorineural hearing loss later in life.

B. Rubella
Congenital rubella can cause similar signs but is often associated with cataracts and congenital heart disease as well as deafness; congenital rubella is extremely rare in the UK since the MMR vaccine was introduced, and all mothers are screened for rubella antibodies.

C. Syphilis
This is unlikely because mothers in the UK are screened for syphilis infection, and we know that this mother's screening bloods were normal.

D. Toxoplasmosis
Babies with toxoplasmosis can have some of the features described, with the addition of intracranial calcification, hydrocephalus, and retinopathy, but this infection is rare in the UK.

E. Varicella zoster
Babies whose mothers develop chickenpox in the first 20 weeks of pregnancy are at risk of severe scarring of the skin, and possibly ocular and neurological damage. However, this is rare.

10.8
D. 7 ⊘
Correct. He scores 2 each for a heart rate >100 beats/min and regular respirations, but only 1 each for some hypotonia and flexion of his limbs, a grimace but no cry, and although his body is pink, his extremities are blue.

10.9
A. Anaemia
This baby has intrauterine growth restriction. These babies are at risk of polycythaemia rather than anaemia.

B. Congenital cardiac abnormality
Congenital cardiac anomalies are not caused by intrauterine growth restriction.

C. Group B streptococcus infection
This baby has intrauterine growth restriction. However, this does not increase the baby's risk of Group B streptococcus infection compared with babies of normal weight.

D. Hypoglycaemia ⊘
Correct. The baby has intrauterine growth restriction. These babies are liable to hypoglycaemia from poor fat and glycogen stores.

E. Hypercalcaemia
This baby has intrauterine growth restriction. These babies are at risk of hypocalcaemia rather than hypercalcaemia.

10.10
A. Cystic fibrosis
This is now screened for in the UK.

B. Duchenne muscular dystrophy ⊘
Correct. This is not routinely screened for. Screening with creatine kinase measurement is unreliable at this age, with many false-positive and false-negative results, and there is insufficient evidence of long-term benefit of diagnosis in the newborn period.

C. Hypothyroidism
Thyroid function is screened. As this is with TSH in the UK, it may miss the rare cases of central hypothyroidism.

D. Phenylketonuria
This was the initial disorder screened for and was called the Guthrie test.

E. Sickle cell disease
This forms part of the newborn screen in the UK.

10.11
A. Congenital rubella syndrome
Characteristic clinical features are not present in this baby.

B. Hypoxic-ischaemic encephalopathy
This could cause some of these neurological abnormalities, but sneezing and yawning and satisfactory condition at birth (good Apgar scores) are against this diagnosis.

C. Fetal alcohol syndrome
These infants have severe growth restriction and have characteristic facies.

D. Kernicterus
Kernicterus is unlikely as severe jaundice is absent.

E. Maternal opiate use ⊘
Correct. The clinical features are consistent with neonatal abstinence syndrome.

10.12
A. Breastfeeding is contra-indicated
Antibodies acquired via breast milk are important for an infant's immunity, although they will not protect against this episode of varicella.

B. Neonatal infection is unlikely due to transplacentally acquired antibodies
The mother is unlikely to have antibodies to varicella, because she herself has developed chickenpox.

C. Reassure and discharge home asking mother to return if the baby develops symptoms
The infant is at risk of morbidity and mortality if discharged home. This advice would be inappropriate.

D. The infant's varicella antibody status should be checked
It is unlikely that the mother will have any antibodies to varicella, as she herself has developed chickenpox. Therefore, transplacental transfer of antibodies cannot have occurred, and the infant will not be immune to varicella.

E. There is a significant risk of serious neonatal infection ⊘
Correct. If the mother develops chickenpox from 5 days before until 5 days after delivery, there will be insufficient time for protective antibodies to develop and be transferred to the infant. A quarter of such infants become infected, with a significant mortality.

Answers: Extended Matching

10.13.1
C. Erythema toxicum
Erythema toxicum or neonatal urticaria is an extremely common rash and appears at day 2–3 of age. It is usually concentrated on the trunk and comes and goes at different sites. The fluid within the papules contains eosinophils.

10.13.2
I. Port wine stain (naevus flammeus)
This is a port wine stain. It is due to a vascular malformation of the capillaries in the dermis. If along the distribution of the trigeminal nerve, it may be associated with intracranial vascular anomalies.

10.13.3
E. Milia
Milia are white pimples on the nose and cheeks. They are due to the retention of keratin and sebaceous material in the pilaceous follicles.

10.13.4
J. Strawberry naevus (cavernous haemangioma)
They are not usually present at birth, but appear in the first month of life. They are more common in preterm infants. They increase in size until 3–9 months of age and then gradually regress.

10.13.5
F. Mongolian blue spots
These are blue/black discolorations at the base of the spine and on the buttocks, most commonly found in Asian and African infants. They fade slowly over the first few years of life, and are of no clinical significance.

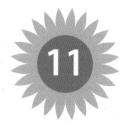

Neonatal medicine

Questions: Single Best Answer

11.1

Natasha, a female infant, is delivered by caesarean section at 32 weeks' gestation because of maternal pre-eclampsia. Her birth weight is 1.9 kg. No resuscitation is required. At 2 hours of age she develops respiratory distress, with a respiratory rate of 70 breaths/min, grunting respirations, and indrawing of her rib cage. Respiratory support with CPAP (continuous positive airway pressure) and 45% oxygen is required. A chest X-ray is taken at 4 hours of age, and is shown (Fig. 11.1).

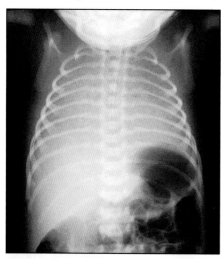

Figure 11.1

What is the most likely reason that this baby needs oxygen therapy and respiratory support?

Select one answer only.

A. Aspiration of meconium has resulted in lung collapse
B. Blood is still flowing from the pulmonary artery to the aorta as in the fetal circulation
C. The alveoli still contain fluid
D. The chest wall and ribs are too compliant
E. There is ventilation-perfusion mismatch from surfactant deficiency

11.2

Robert is a full term male infant, born 10 hours ago. His mother is blood group O rhesus positive and her membranes ruptured 2 days before delivery. He is breastfeeding well but the midwife noticed he looks jaundiced. On examination the baby is clinically well but markedly jaundiced.

What investigation should be performed first?

Select one answer only.

A. Bilirubin level
B. Blood culture
C. Blood group
D. Congenital infection screen
E. Direct antibody test

11.3

You are asked to review a newborn baby who is only 24 hours old and has developed very swollen eyelids with a purulent discharge.

What management is required?

Select one answer only.

A. Clean with cool boiled water
B. Intravenous antibiotics
C. Oral antibiotics
D. Reassure that it will resolve spontaneously
E. Topical antibiotic therapy

11.4

Isabelle was born at term weighing 4 kg. At 6 hours of age she was noted to be breathing fast and have a low temperature. She was born by normal vaginal delivery and the membranes had ruptured 24 hours previously. Isabelle has not breastfed since birth and has had one vomit. On examination, she is lethargic and her core temperature is 35.5°C. She has a respiratory rate of 90 breaths/min, her central capillary refill time is 4 seconds, pulse 180/min and oxygen saturation is 89% in air.

Her chest X-ray shows consolidation at the right base.

What is the most likely causative organism for her infection?

Select one answer only.

A. *Escherichia coli (E. coli)*
B. Group B streptococcus
C. Herpes simplex virus (HSV) infection
D. *Listeria monocytogenes*
E. *Staphylococcus aureus*

11.5

James was born at 39 weeks' gestation by elective caesarean section because of pre-eclampsia. His birth weight was 3.7 kg. His mother breastfed him as soon as she had recovered from the general anaesthetic. He fed well but is vomiting after every feed. He is now 18 hours old and after the last 2 feeds he 'vomited everything up' and it was greenish in colour. On examination his temperature is 36.5°C and he is alert and hungry.

His abdomen is not distended. He has not yet passed meconium.

What is the most likely diagnosis?

Select one answer only.

A. Duodenal atresia
B. Hirschprung disease
C. Meconium ileus
D. Neonatal sepsis
E. Pyloric stenosis

11.6

Aaron was born at term, birth weight 3.2 kg. He is now 2 weeks old, and his mother is concerned that his umbilicus looks abnormal. A photo is shown in Fig. 11.2.

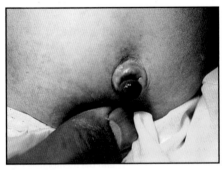

Figure 11.2

Select the most likely diagnosis.

Select one answer only.

A. Exomphalos
B. Gastroschisis
C. Umbilical granuloma
D. Umbilical hernia
E. Umbilical infection (omphalitis)

Questions: Extended Matching

11.7

The following is a list of possible diagnoses(A–L). For each clinical case described below select the most likely diagnosis. Each answer may be used once, more than once, or not at all.

A. Anaemia
B. Bronchopulmonary dysplasia (BPD)
C. Coarctation of the aorta
D. Diaphragmatic hernia
E. Heart failure
F. Meconium aspiration
G. Persistent pulmonary hypertension of the newborn (PPHN)
H. Pneumonia
I. Pneumothorax
J. Respiratory distress syndrome
K. Tracheo-oesphageal fistula
L. Transient tachypnoea of the newborn

11.7.1

Mohammed was born at term, weighing 3 kg. He is 6 hours old and on the postnatal ward with his mother, who has asked the midwife to review him as he is breathing very quickly. Mohammed did not breathe well immediately after birth and needed mask ventilation to establish breathing. By 5 minutes of age he was crying and was wrapped and handed to his mother. On examination he is breathing at 64 breaths/min, and there is mild chest recession. Breath sounds on the left side are reduced compared with the right. His oxygen saturation is 95%. The chest X-ray is shown (Fig. 11.3).

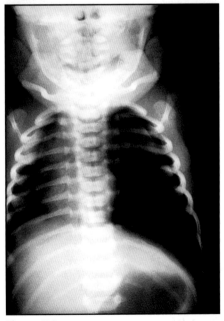

Figure 11.3

11.7.2

Sabrina was born at 37 weeks' gestation, birth weight 2.8 kg. She was noted by the midwife to be breathing very fast at 2 hours of age. On examination she is breathing at 72 breaths/min and has moderate chest recession. The heart sounds are difficult to hear on the left and her apex beat is palpable on the right side of the chest. A chest X-ray is taken (Fig. 11.4).

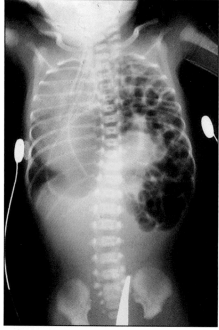

Figure 11.4

11.7.3

Thomas, a baby boy with a birth weight of 875 g at 28 weeks' gestation required artificial ventilation for 2 weeks. At 10 weeks of age he still needs additional oxygen via nasal cannulae. This is his chest X-ray (Fig. 11.5)

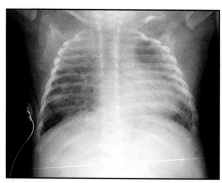

Figure 11.5

11.8

The following is a list of diagnoses that are associated with jaundice in the newborn period. For each of the following scenarios pick the most likely cause of the jaundice. Each answer may be used once, more than once, or not at all.

A. ABO incompatibility
B. Biliary atresia
C. Breast milk jaundice
D. Congenital hypothyroidism
E. Congenital infection with cytomegalovirus
F. Crigler–Najjar syndrome
G. G6PD deficiency
H. Physiological jaundice
I. Rhesus haemolytic disease
J. Sepsis
K. Urinary tract infection

11.8.1

Stewart is a full-term baby boy, born 16 hours ago. His mother is blood group O rhesus positive. The baby is breastfeeding well but the midwife has noticed he looks jaundiced. On examination the baby is clinically well. His bilirubin was 150 μmol/L at 10 hours and he was started on intensive phototherapy. Six hours later his bilirubin is 250 μmol/L. Stewart's blood group was identified as group A rhesus positive.

11.8.2

Alfie is a 3-week-old male infant whose mother is concerned that his stools are pale. He is breastfed. On examination he is jaundiced, has mild hepatomegaly and has only just regained his birthweight.

11.8.3

Poppy is 2 weeks old and is breastfed. She is thriving but is jaundiced. The midwife does a bilirubin which is moderately raised at 170 μmol/L, and is nearly all unconjugated. A urine dipstick is negative.

11.8.4

Dimitri is 20 hours old and is noted to be markedly jaundiced, needing intensive phototherapy. Maternal blood is group A rhesus positive. His blood group is group A rhesus positive. He has been breastfeeding well. On examination he is markedly jaundiced, but is alert and active.

11.9

The following is a list (A–L) of diagnoses that are associated with respiratory distress in the newborn period. For each of the following scenarios pick the most likely cause of the jaundice. Each answer may be used once, more than once or not at all.

For each of the scenarios, choose the most likely diagnosis from the list.

A. Anaemia
B. Bronchopulmonary dysplasia (BPD)
C. Coarctation of the aorta
D. Diaphragmatic hernia
E. Heart failure
F. Meconium aspiration
G. Persistent pulmonary hypertension of the newborn
H. Pneumonia
I. Pneumothorax
J. Respiratory distress syndrome
K. Tracheo-oesophageal fistula
L. Transient tachypnoea of the newborn

11.9.1

Rebecca was born 48 hours ago at term. She weighed 3.2 kg. You are asked to review her on the postnatal ward as she is breathing very quickly. She is not feeding. On examination she is breathing at 68 breaths/min and has mild chest recession. She looks unwell. You cannot confidently feel her femoral pulses. Her oxygen saturation is 85% in air.

11.9.2

Zak, a full-term male infant, with a birth weight of 3.7 kg, is born by elective caesarean section. His mother was well during pregnancy and had a normal blood glucose screen. Zak becomes tachypnoeic with indrawing between his ribs at 2 hours of age. Examination is otherwise normal. A chest X-ray looks normal.

Answers: Single Best Answer

11.1
A. Aspiration of meconium has resulted in lung collapse
Meconium aspiration is associated with term or post-term infants. There are patchy changes on chest X-ray (CXR).

B. Blood is still flowing from the pulmonary artery to the aorta as in the fetal circulation
Some blood may 'shunt' across a PDA (persistent ductus arteriosus) but this would usually flow from the high pressure aorta into the pulmonary artery as pulmonary vascular resistance should drop after birth and inflation of the lungs.

C. The alveoli still contain fluid
Retention of a small amount of fluid is common and results in transient tachypnoea of the newborn.

D. The chest wall and ribs are too compliant
The ribs are compliant but this is not the main reason for respiratory distress.

E. **There is ventilation-perfusion mismatch from surfactant deficiency** ⊘
Correct. Surfactant deficiency is common in preterm infants. This results in alveolar collapse which in turn results in areas of lung being perfused but not ventilated. The CXR appearance here is typical with a diffuse granular or 'ground glass' appearance.

11.2
A. **Bilirubin level** ⊘
Correct. Jaundice starting at less than 24 hours of age is most likely due to haemolysis and may rapidly rise to dangerously high levels. It needs urgent assessment and close monitoring. The most urgent investigation is to measure the bilirubin level, as this will determine the management required.

B. Blood culture
Blood cultures are taken to exclude infection but do not influence immediate management.

C. Blood group
Blood group will inform if ABO or Rhesus incompatibility is a likely cause but will not influence immediate management.

D. Congenital infection screen
Congenital infection can cause early jaundice but there are usually clinical features and the jaundice is mild.

E. Direct antibody test
Direct antibody test is positive with rhesus disease and ABO incompatibility.

11.3
A. Clean with cool boiled water
The eyes should be cleaned and carefully examined but also treated pending the results of any swabs.

B. **Intravenous antibiotics** ⊘
Correct. Purulent discharge and eyelid swelling in the first 48 hours of life must be taken seriously. This should be treated promptly, e.g. with a third-generation cephalosporin intravenously, as permanent loss of vision can occur. The most common cause of severe neonatal purulent conjunctivitis is *Chlamydia trachomatis,* but gonococcus may also be the cause.

C. Oral antibiotics
Oral antibiotic absorption in the newborn is highly variable and therefore cannot be relied upon to treat this (or other) infections.

D. Reassure that it will resolve spontaneously
Whilst incomplete canalization of the nasolacrimal duct commonly leads to sticky eyes, the discharge is rarely purulent and the eyes are not swollen.

E. Topical antibiotic therapy
Topical antibiotic therapy is often prescribed for a sticky eye in older infants and children but is insufficient in this situation.

11.4
A. *Escherichia coli (E. coli)*
An important cause of neonatal sepsis but not as common as Group B streptococcus. Antibiotic regimens to treat newborn infants must cover this organism though.

B. **Group B streptococcus** ⊘
Correct. Isabelle is most likely to have early-onset sepsis and this can be caused by infection in the chest, urine or cerebrospinal fluid (meningitis). The most common organism causing early-onset sepsis in the UK is Group B *streptococcus.*
Listeria monocytogenes, E. coli, and *Staphylococcus aureus* may cause early-onset sepsis, but are less common causes in the UK.

C. Herpes simplex virus (HSV) infection
HSV infection in the neonate is rare but very serious when it occurs. It can present with localized lesions, encephalitis, or disseminated disease. Treatment is with intravenous aciclovir. Primary maternal HSV infection may not be diagnosed at delivery. Skin lesions may not be present.

D. *Listeria monocytogenes*
An important cause of neonatal sepsis and meningitis but rare in the UK. Antibiotic regimens to treat newborn infants must cover this organism though.

E. *Staphylococcus aureus*
A common cause of skin infection but can cause sepsis or staphylococcal scalded skin syndrome in the newborn. Blistering rashes or inflammation around the umbilicus increase the likelihood of this infection.

11.5
A. Duodenal atresia ⊘
Correct. This is the most likely cause of persistent bilious vomiting on the 1st day of life. Malrotation and volvulus can also cause this presentation, but the vomit may contain blood and the abdomen may be tender. A plain abdominal X-ray would be helpful as it may show the classic 'double bubble'.

B. Hirschprung disease
Affects the rectum and sometimes the colon, therefore causes distal bowel obstruction causing marked abdominal distension.

C. Meconium ileus
Affects the lower ileum, so there would be abdominal obstruction and therefore distension.

D. Neonatal sepsis
Neonatal sepsis can cause vomiting, which is sometimes slightly bile-stained, but there are no risk factors from labour and delivery, and no other features on clinical examination.

E. Pyloric stenosis
In pyloric stenosis the vomit is not bile-stained as the obstruction is above the ampulla of Vater and it presents at about 6 weeks of age.

11.6
A. Exomphalos
In exomphalos the abdominal contents protrude through the umbilical ring, covered by the amniotic membrane and peritoneum.

B. Gastroschisis
In gastroschisis the bowel protrudes through a defect in the anterior abdominal wall adjacent to the umbilicus.

C. Umbilical granuloma ⊘
Correct. In umbilical granuloma there is a pink, pedunculated lesion of granulation tissue as shown here.

D. Umbilical hernia
In umbilical hernia there is protrusion of the umbilicus. These are common and resolve spontaneously.

E. Umbilical infection (omphalitis)
In umbilical infection (omphalitis) there is redness of the skin surrounding the umbilicus, with spread of the redness onto the anterior abdominal wall (umbilical flare). Sometimes there is purulent discharge, although an umbilical granuloma can also be 'sticky' as it produces mucus.

Answers: Extended Matching

11.7.1
I. Pneumothorax
This may have been spontaneous, but the risk is increased by the positive pressure ventilation during resuscitation. Nonetheless, a pneumothorax may occur spontaneously in 1–2% of newborn infants. The reduced breath sounds are because of the pneumothorax. The diagnosis is confirmed on chest X-ray, with hypertranslucency on the left, the left lung edge is visible, and the mediastinum is displaced to the right.

11.7.2
D. Diaphragmatic hernia
The chest X-ray shows loops of bowel in the left chest and there is displacement of the mediastinum

11.7.3
B. Bronchopulmonary dysplasia (BPD)
This is the name used for infants born preterm who still have an oxygen requirement at a postmenstrual age of 36 weeks. The X-ray characteristically shows widespread areas of opacification and cystic changes.

11.8.1
A. ABO incompatibility
This is now more common than rhesus haemolytic disease. Most ABO antibodies are IgM and do not cross the placenta, but some group O women have an IgG anti-A-haemolysin in the blood which can cross the placenta and haemolyses the red cells of a group A infant. Occasionally, group B infants are affected by anti-B haemolysins.

11.8.2
B. Biliary atresia
Conjugated hyperbilirubinaemia is suggested by the pale stools accompanying his jaundice. His urine will be dark but this may not be recognized. There are other causes of conjugated hyperbilirubinaemia in infants of this age but it is important to diagnose biliary atresia as early as possible, as early surgery improves prognosis.

11.8.3
C. Breast milk jaundice
In most infants with prolonged neonatal jaundice, the hyperbilirubinaemia is unconjugated, but this needs to be confirmed on laboratory testing. In prolonged unconjugated hyperbilirubinaemia, 'breast milk jaundice' is the most common cause, affecting up to 15% of healthy breastfed infants; the jaundice gradually fades and disappears by 4–5 weeks of age.

11.8.4
G. G6PD deficiency
Dimitri has severe jaundice at less than 24 hours of age, therefore it is likely to be haemolytic. His

mother's and his blood group, A and rhesus positive, exclude rhesus disease and ABO incompatibility. His parents' Mediterranean origin is compatible with G6PD deficiency, a common and important cause of haemolytic jaundice worldwide.

11.9.1
C. Coarctation of the aorta
The absence of femoral pulses should always suggest that there is coarctation of the aorta. Her left brachial pulse will also be difficult to palpate. Heart failure develops when the ductus arteriosus closes as this is a classic 'duct-dependent' lesion.

11.9.2
L. Transient tachypnoea of the newborn
The most common cause of respiratory distress in a term infant. It is due to a delay in the resorption of lung liquid – an increased risk following caesarean section, as the babies have not had to undergo the same physical and physiological stressors as those who pass through the birth canal.

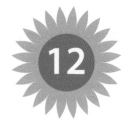

Growth and puberty

Questions: Single Best Answer

12.1
Janine, a 9-month-old female infant, is seen by her family doctor because of concern that she is not growing fast enough. She is only on the 5th centile for height and 2nd centile for weight.

What is the greatest influence on her growth rate at her age?

Select one answer only.

A. Genes
B. Growth hormone
C. Nutrition
D. Oestrogen
E. Testosterone

12.2
John, a 3-year-old boy, is referred to paediatric outpatients because of concern about the development of pubic and axillary hair. His testes are 1.5 ml in size (prepubertal). His blood pressure is 100/75 mmHg. Gonadotrophin levels are normal for a prepubertal boy (undetectable) but his bone age is 5 years.

What is the most likely cause of his early pubertal development?

Select one answer only.

A. Adrenal tumour
B. Brain tumour
C. Idiopathic precocious puberty
D. Prader–Willi syndrome
E. Testicular tumour

12.3
Chelsea, a 7-year-old girl, is brought by her mother to the paediatric clinic. Her mother is concerned about Chelsea's early development of puberty. Chelsea has started to develop breasts and, more recently, some pubic hair. On examination she has breast development stage 3 and pubic hair development stage 2 (see Fig. 12.5, Illustrated Textbook of Paediatrics). She has not started her periods, but has had a growth spurt recently. An ultrasound of her pelvis shows multicystic ovaries and enlarging uterus.

What is the most likely cause of her early pubertal development?

Select one answer only.

A. Brain tumour
B. Congenital adrenal hyperplasia
C. Idiopathic precocious puberty
D. Ovarian tumour
E. Turner syndrome

12.4
Sophia, an 18-month-old girl, is brought to outpatients by her mother, who is very worried as she has developed breasts. She is otherwise well and has been growing normally. On examination she has breast development stage 3 (BIII) but no pubic or axillary hair. Her bone age is 20 months.

What is the most likely cause of her early pubertal development?

Select one answer only.

A. Brain tumour
B. Congenital adrenal hyperplasia
C. Idiopathic precocious puberty
D. Premature thelarche
E. Premature pubarche

12.5
Tom, a 7-year-old boy, is referred by his general practitioner with concerns about his growth. He is an adopted child and no details are available about his biological father although his biological mother was 'of average height'. Physical examination reveals a happy and playful boy with no dysmorphic features. His height is 110 cm which is just below the 0.4th centile. His weight is on the 0.4th centile. He has a normal physical examination.

What is the most likely cause for his short stature?

Select one answer only.

A. Achondroplasia
B. Constitutional delay of growth and puberty
C. Familial short stature
D. Growth hormone deficiency
E. Vitamin D deficiency

Questions: Extended Matching

12.6

The following (A–M) is a list of investigations for children referred with short stature. From the following clinical scenarios pick the investigation which is most likely lead to a correct diagnosis. Each answer may be used once, more than once, or not at all.

A. Bone age (wrist X-ray)
B. Coeliac screen
C. C-reactive protein (CRP) and erythrocyte sedimentation rate (ESR)
D. Creatinine and electrolytes
E. Full blood count
F. Growth hormone provocation tests
G. Insulin-like growth factor-1 (IGF-1)
H. Karyotype
I. MRI scan of the brain
J. Skeletal survey
K. Thyroid stimulating hormone (TSH)
L. Ultrasound scan of the uterus
M. Vitamin D levels

12.6.1

May, a 14-year-old girl, is referred by her school nurse because she is found to be below the 0.4th centile for height. He mother is 167 cm tall and father is 175 cm tall. She was born at term, birth weight 3.2 kg. She says she has always been the shortest in the class. Physical examination reveals a girl in the early stages of puberty. Her previous history is unremarkable. Her blood pressure is 135/65 mmHg.

12.6.2

Eleanor, a 7-year-old girl, is referred because of short stature. She is on the 5th centile for height and 25th centile for weight. Her growth chart shows that 9 months previously her height and weight were on the 15th centile. Her mother says that she has become lethargic, her school work has deteriorated and that she now refuses to do sport.

12.6.3

Jake, a 5-year-old boy with Down syndrome has a check-up with his general practitioner. He is short but until 6 months ago was following his growth centiles. You note that his height has dropped one centile line and his weight two centile lines. His mother reports that he has become very irritable and difficult to manage. On direct questioning, his appetite has deteriorated, with meal times becoming problematic.

Answers: Single Best Answer

12.1.
A. Genes
Genes are important but without adequate nutrition a child's growth potential will not be achieved. Genetic influences begin to affect growth mostly after the 1st year of life.

B. Growth hormone
Growth hormone is particularly important in determining growth after infancy and continues to exert an effect until growth ceases.

C. Nutrition ⊘
Correct. Along with good health, happiness and thyroid hormones, infant growth (from birth to 12 months of age) is most dependent on good nutrition. Growth in the 1st year of life contributes about 15% to final adult height.

D. Oestrogen
The sex hormones cause the back to lengthen and boost growth hormone secretion. This occurs during the pubertal growth spurt.

E. Testosterone
The sex hormones cause the back to lengthen and boost growth hormone secretion. This occurs during the pubertal growth spurt.

12.2.
A. Adrenal tumour ⊘
Correct. Premature sexual development in boys is uncommon and usually has an organic (rather than constitutional or familial) cause. With his prepubertal testes, hypertension and normal gonadotrophin levels, the abnormality is likely to be in his adrenal glands.

B. Brain tumour
John has prepubertal testes; therefore he does not have true precocious puberty and the cause is not likely to be central.

C. Idiopathic precocious puberty
He has prepubertal testes so does not have precocious puberty.

D. Prader–Willi syndrome
Boys with Prader–Willi syndrome have delayed puberty.

E. Testicular tumour
John has prepubertal testes; therefore, he does not have precocious puberty and the cause is not likely to be coming from his testes.

12.3.
A. Brain tumour
You would be more worried about the likelihood of a brain tumour if this was a boy showing signs of early puberty.

B. Congenital adrenal hyperplasia
In congenital adrenal hyperplasia, the sequence of pubertal changes is abnormal, with isolated pubic hair and virilisation of genitalia.

C. Idiopathic precocious puberty ⊘
Correct. Precocious puberty in females is usually due to premature onset of normal puberty. The sequence of puberty in this child is normal and there is also been an associated growth spurt, which makes an idiopathic cause for the precocious puberty more likely.

D. Ovarian tumour
The pelvic ultrasound findings are consistent with premature onset of normal puberty.

E. Turner syndrome
Turner syndrome is associated with delayed rather than precocious puberty.

12.4.
A. Brain tumour
A brain tumour is unlikely as she has isolated breast development.

B. Congenital adrenal hyperplasia
Congenital adrenal hyperplasia would cause premature pubarche rather than isolated breast development.

C. Idiopathic precocious puberty
Sophia does not have precocious puberty because she does not have axillary or pubic hair, nor has she had a growth spurt.

D. Premature thelarche ⊘
Correct. Sophia has breast development and no other signs of puberty. She has premature thelarche.

E. Premature pubarche
She has not developed pubic or axillary hair.

12.5.
A. Achondroplasia
He has no dysmporhic features. There would be obvious disproportion with shorter limbs if this was the diagnosis.

B. Constitutional delay of growth and puberty
Tom is too young to present with this. His pubertal growth spurt would not be expected until the second decade of life.

C. Familial short stature ⊘
Correct. Most short children have short parents and fall within the centile target range allowing for midparental height. Care needs to be taken, though, that both the child and a parent do not have an inherited growth disorder, such as a skeletal dysplasia.

D. Growth hormone deficiency
It is possible, but not the most likely cause of short stature. Careful re-evaluation and assessment of the growth velocity will be helpful.

E. Vitamin D deficiency
It is unlikely to be the cause of growth failure without other signs of rickets (swollen wrists, bent legs).

Answers: Extended Matching

12.6.1
H. Karyotype
Turner syndrome needs to be excluded as she has always been short. The elevated blood pressure may be because of an undetected coarctation of the aorta which is associated with the syndrome.

12.6.2
K. Thyroid stimulating hormone (TSH)
Her height has stopped increasing and she has put on weight. This suggests an endocrine problem. Her clinical symptoms suggest hypothyroidism.

12.6.3
B. Coeliac screen
Children with Down syndrome are at increased risk. He is also at increased risk of hypothyroidism, but his decreased appetite, irritability and weight loss are characteristic of coeliac disease.

Nutrition

Questions: Single Best Answer

13.1
Sunit, a 13-month-old boy, presents with faltering growth. He is still entirely breastfed. On examination, he is miserable and his wrist is shown in Fig. 13.1a. An X-ray is taken of his wrist is shown in Fig. 13.1b.

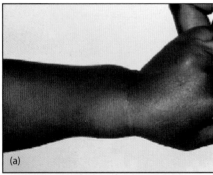

(a)

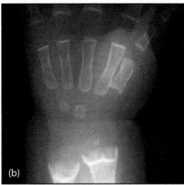

(b)

Figure 13.1 a) Courtesy of Nick Shaw.

What is the most likely diagnosis?

Select one answer only.

A. Vitamin A deficiency
B. Vitamin B1 deficiency
C. Vitamin D deficiency
D. Vitamin E deficiency
E. Vitamin K deficiency

13.2
Sarah, a 9-year-old girl, is referred by the school nurse to the paediatric clinic because of her weight. She weighs 43 kg (98th centile) and is 141 cm tall (91st centile). She has followed her height centiles for the last 9 months but her weight centile has increased. Her body mass index is on the 97th centile. Her mother reports that she hardly eats at all and when she does she has a very healthy diet.

Which of the following statements is most likely to be correct?

Select one answer only.

A. A calorie-restricted diet is the treatment of choice
B. Sarah's adrenocortical axis should be checked to exclude Cushing syndrome
C. Sarah has a higher risk of an abnormal lipid profile and raised blood pressure in adult life
D. Sarah is obese
E. Sarah's main problem is that she has a low metabolic rate

13.3
Which of the following term newborns has the lowest risk of cardiovascular disease in later life?

Select one answer only.

A. 1.8 kg
B. 2.1 kg
C. 2.4 kg
D. 3.9 kg
E. 4.6 kg

13.4
A mother asks you whether there are any disadvantages to breastfeeding. Although you would prefer to inform her about the many advantages of breastfeeding, you wish to answer her question honestly. Which of the following is most likely to be a true potential disadvantage?

Select one answer only.

A. Breastfeeding will reduce her chance of having more children
B. The absence of cow's milk protein in breast milk increases the risk that the child will develop milk allergy at weaning
C. The higher interferon level in breast milk increases the risk of severe bronchiolitis in children who develop respiratory syncytial virus infection
D. The lower vitamin K concentration in breast milk can result in life-threatening bleeding
E. The strong bond developed during breastfeeding will prevent paternal bonding

13.5
Anil is a 2½-year-old boy who lives in India and attends the local health clinic near their village for a routine check. Both his parents are subsistence farmers. He is asymptomatic. On examination, he is very thin but his hair and skin appear normal and there is no oedema or other clinical abnormalities. His height is on the 5th centile but his weight is well below the 0.4th centile (z-score between −2 and −3 below the median).

What is the most likely diagnosis?

Select one answer only.

A. Kwashiorkor
B. Marasmus
C. Normal child
D. Rickets
E. Severe gastro-oesophageal reflux

13.6
Harry is a 13-year-old boy who attends the paediatric clinic because of obesity. His height is on the 98th centile and his weight is above the 99.6th centile.

Which of the following is least likely to be associated with obesity?

Select one answer only.

A. Asthma
B. Hypertension
C. Low self-esteem
D. Slipped upper femoral epiphysis
E. Type 1 diabetes

Questions: Extended Matching

13.7
For each of the following patients with nutritional problems select the most likely diagnosis from the list (A–J) below. Each option may be used once, more than once, or not at all.

A. Cow's milk protein allergy
B. Cystic fibrosis
C. Kwashiorkor
D. Marasmus
E. Normal
F. Obesity
G. Vitamin A deficiency
H. Vitamin C deficiency
I. Vitamin D deficiency
J. Vitamin K deficiency

13.7.1
Ahmed is an 18-month-old Pakistani boy who was born in the UK with a weight of 3.2 kg. He is on a mixed diet. His height is on the 10th centile and his weight is on the 0.4th centile. He is noted to be miserable. On examination, his wrists also feel wider than normal.

13.7.2
Harry is a 3-week-old infant who has been exclusively breastfed by his mother. He was born at home as his mother wanted 'everything to be natural' and declined all interventions. His birthweight was 3.4 kg. He presents to the hospital with severe rectal bleeding and shock.

13.7.3
Jonas is an 18-month-old black African boy in KwaZulu Natal, South Africa. He was born weighing 3.2 kg. He was breastfed until 9 months of age when his sibling was born. He now mainly eats the traditional maize-based porridge, which is grown on the family farm. His weight is just below the 0.4th centile. He looks thin but has a distended abdomen. There is oedema around his eyes and the top of his feet. His hair has a red tinge.

13.7.4
Jamie is a 5-month-old male infant who was born with a weight of 3.5 kg (25th centile). He was initially breastfed and was growing well. His mother developed mastitis and so he was changed to formula milk feeds. He now weighs 5.0 kg (<0.4th centile). He has frequent loose stools and eczema.

13.7.5
Tanya, an 11-month-old Caucasian girl, is being monitored by her health visitor. Her birthweight was 2.4 kg (0.4th centile) and she has remained on the 2nd centile, now weighing 7.0 kg. Her mother is on the 5th centile and her father is on the 40th centile for height. She is well, has a good appetite and has never needed to visit her doctor. She has no abnormal signs on examination and her development is normal.

Answers: Single Best Answer

13.1

A. Vitamin A deficiency
Clinical manifestations of vitamin A deficiency include eye damage from corneal scarring and impairment of mucosal function and immunity. These complications are seen in low-resource countries.

B. Vitamin B1 deficiency
Thiamine (vitamin B1) is a cofactor for many enzymes. Clinical features include cardiac features (e.g. heart failure) and neurological features (e.g. polyneuropathy).

C. Vitamin D deficiency ⊘
Correct. He has vitamin D deficiency resulting in rickets. This classically causes bowing of the legs but now more often presents with poor growth. The ends of the radius and ulna, as shown on the x-ray of the wrists, (and the tibia and fibula at the ankles) are expanded and rarefied and cup shaped. At 13 months of age, breast milk alone does not provide adequate intake of vitamin D.

D. Vitamin E deficiency
Vitamin E deficiency is rare. It is a fat-soluble vitamin and can therefore result from severe fat malabsorption, e.g. abetalipoproteinemia or in cystic fibrosis. Individuals with CF are routinely prescribed vitamin supplements to counter these problems. Vitamin E deficiency causes a neuropathy and ataxia.

E. Vitamin K deficiency
Vitamin K deficiency affects the clotting factors II, VII, IX, and X. It is a fat-soluble vitamin, and can be due to fat malabsorption or present as haemorrhagic disease of the newborn.

13.2

A. A calorie-restricted diet is the treatment of choice
The current recommendation is for a well-balanced healthy diet with increased physical activity rather than calorie restriction alone. Many surveys of food intake of overweight children show that the quantity of food they consume is no greater than normal weight children.

B. Sarah's adrenocortical axis should be checked to exclude Cushing syndrome
Cushing syndrome is rare and associated with a failure of linear growth.

C. Sarah has an increased risk of an abnormal lipid profile and raised blood pressure in adult life ⊘
Correct. Sarah is overweight [body mass index (BMI) > 91st centile] rather than obese (BMI > 98th centile). It places her at increased risk of an abnormal lipid profile and raised blood pressure in adult life unless action is taken.

D. Sarah is obese
For clinical use, obese children are those with a BMI above the 98th centile of the UK 1990 reference chart for age and sex. Sarah is overweight (BMI > 91st centile).

E. Sarah's main problem is that she has a low metabolic rate
In most cases, obesity results from an increased intake of energy-dense foods and reduced exercise.

13.3

A. Birthweight 1.8 kg
Evidence suggests that undernutrition in utero resulting in growth restriction is associated with an increased incidence of coronary heart disease, stroke, type 2 diabetes, and hypertension in later life.

B. Birthweight 2.1 kg
The risk is significantly higher than babies born weighing between 3.9 kg and 4.3 kg.

C. Birthweight 2.4 kg
The risk is still significantly higher than babies born weighing between 3.9 kg and 4.3 kg.

D. Birthweight 3.9 kg ⊘
Correct. The lowest risk of cardiovascular disease, almost half that of babies born weighing less than 2.5 kg. This is the Barker hypothesis – see Figure 13.3 in Illustrated Textbook of Paediatrics.

E. Birthweight 4.6 kg
The risk appears to increase again for very heavy babies and this may be related to factors such as maternal diabetes.

13.4

A. Breastfeeding will reduce her chance of having more children
Breastfeeding leads to an increased period between children on a population basis. However, it is not an effective form of contraception, and does not decrease fertility.

B. The absence of cow's milk protein in breast milk increases the risk that the child will develop milk allergy at weaning
Cow's milk allergy is more commonly seen in bottle-fed infants. However, a small amount of milk protein does pass into the breast milk and cow's milk allergy occurs in up to 1 in 200 breastfed babies. Exposure to small amounts of cow's milk protein probably lowers rather than increases the risk.

C. The higher interferon level in breast milk increases the risk of severe bronchiolitis in children who develop respiratory syncytial virus infection

Interferon is present in breast milk and has an antiviral property. Breastfeeding does not lead to a more severe bronchiolitis.

D. The lower vitamin K concentration in breast milk can result in life-threatening bleeding ⊘
Correct. The vitamin K concentration in breast milk is lower. There is insufficient vitamin K in breast milk to reliably prevent haemorrhagic disease of the newborn. This risk is minimized by giving prophylactic vitamin K.

E. The strong bond developed during breast-feeding will prevent paternal bonding
Breastfeeding enhances mother–child relationship but it does not decrease paternal–child bonding.

13.5
A. Kwashiorkor
Kwashiorkor is another manifestation of severe protein malnutrition, but oedema is present.

B. Marasmus ⊘
Correct. In marasmus there is severe protein–energy malnutrition. Oedema is absent.

C. Normal child
Anil is severely underweight.

D. Rickets
Children with rickets can have faltering growth, but they may also have clinical features of rickets: bowing of legs, rachitic rosary, and swelling of ankles and wrists.

E. Severe gastro-oesophageal reflux
There is no history of vomiting.

13.6
A. Asthma
For reasons that are unclear, asthma is more common in obese children and adults.

B. Hypertension
Children who are obese are more likely to develop hypertension.

C. Low self-esteem
Children who are obese are more likely to have low self-esteem.

D. Slipped upper femoral epiphysis
Children who are obese are more likely to develop this complication. This is thought to be

due to increased mechanical stress placed across the space between the upper femoral epiphysis and the femur.

E. Type 1 diabetes ⊘
Correct. Obese children are more likely to have non-insulin dependent diabetes mellitus (type 2 diabetes). Type 1 diabetes is an autoimmune disorder and is not related to a child's weight.

Answers: Extended Matching

13.7.1
I. Vitamin D deficiency
This is more common in children with dark skin. The clinical features of rickets in this child may include bowing of his legs and widening of the wrists. There is increased prevalence of rickets in young children from Southeast Asia living in the UK, from dietary deficiency and inadequate exposure to sunlight.

13.7.2
J. Vitamin K deficiency, causing haemorrhagic disease of the newborn
There is insufficient vitamin K in breast milk to reliably prevent the disorder. Most babies are given prophylactic vitamin K at birth, usually intramuscularly or else orally, but this requires parental consent. Formula feeds are supplemented with vitamin K.

13.7.3
C. Kwashiorkor
He has severe protein malnutrition accompanied by oedema. Because of the oedema, the weight may not be as severely reduced as in marasmus. He has other features of kwashiorkor, the depigmented hair and distended abdomen.

13.7.4
A. Cow's milk protein allergy
He developed faltering growth, loose stools and eczema when changed from breast milk to formula milk, which is based on cow's milk protein.

13.7.5
E. Normal infant
She is growing normally along the 2nd centile for weight, and has no symptoms to suggest an underlying illness. She has short parents and is constitutionally small.

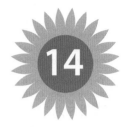

Gastroenterology

Questions: Single Best Answer

14.1

Benjamin is a 6-year-old boy who is seen in the paediatric emergency department. He has been vomiting and has had diarrhoea for 3 days. His stool is watery and foul smelling but has no blood in it. He has not been out of the UK since he was born. Examination reveals mild dehydration but is otherwise normal.

What is the most likely organism that has caused his symptoms?

Select one answer only.

A. *Campylobacter*
B. *Escherichia coli*
C. *Giardia lamblia*
D. Rotavirus
E. *Shigella*

14.2

Emma is an 18-month-old girl who is seen in the outpatient department. She presents with loose stools two to three times each day, with no blood in them. She is generally difficult and it has become a battle to get her to feed. Examination of her abdomen, although difficult due to distress at being examined, is unremarkable apart from being distended. She is not on any medication. Her weight was on the 9th centile and is now below the 0.4th centile.

What is the most likely cause for the weight loss?

Select one answer only.

A. Chronic non-specific diarrhoea
B. Coeliac disease
C. Hirschsprung disease
D. Lactose intolerance
E. Ulcerative colitis

14.3

Rodney, a boisterous 2-year-old, has had diarrhoea for the last 3 months. He produces up to four stools a day, which are loose, brown in colour and usually contain undigested food. The rest of the family are well. He has never been abroad. Examination is normal and his personal child health record shows that he is growing along the 50th centile.

What is the most likely diagnosis?

A. Chronic non-specific diarrhoea
B. Coeliac disease
C. Cow's milk protein allergy
D. Inflammatory bowel disease
E. Lactose intolerance

14.4

Ellie is a 4-year-old girl who has been complaining of pain in her tummy for a month. It is worse when she goes to the toilet; her stools are firm and she opens her bowels only every 2–3 days. She has not had any vomiting. For the last 2 weeks her stools have become loose. On examination she has a mass in the left iliac fossa.

What is the most likely diagnosis?

Select one answer only.

A. Appendix mass
B. Constipation
C. Gastroenteritis
D. Inguinal hernia
E. Wilms tumour

14.5

Aiysha is a 2-month-old baby who is seen in the paediatric outpatient department. She was born at term, weighing 3.5 kg and is breastfed. Her mother is concerned as she has vomited some of the milk after most feeds since birth. She cries when she vomits. She is continuing to grow along the 50th centile.

What is the most likely diagnosis?

Select one answer only.

A. Gastro-oesophageal reflux
B. *Helicobacter pylori* infection

C. Infant colic
D. Overfeeding
E. Pyloric stenosis

14.6

Claire, a 7-year-old girl, has had abdominal pain for the last 6 months. On several occasions it has been sufficiently severe for her to be sent home early from school. The pain happens once or twice a week in the afternoon or early evening. It is periumbilical in nature. It does not wake her at night. She has not had vomiting or diarrhoea. She is growing well. Her examination is normal. Her urine is clear on dipstick testing.

What is the most likely cause for her pain?

Select one answer only.

A. Functional abdominal pain
B. Gastritis
C. Hepatitis A
D. Irritable bowel syndrome
E. Meckel diverticulum

14.7

Ben, aged 9 months, has had a 3 day history of diarrhoea and vomiting. On examination he is found to be quiet but alert, is tachypnoeic, has a tachycardia but normal pulses, dry mouth, no mottling of the skin but reduced skin turgor and a sunken fontanelle. Capillary refill time is 2 seconds. His blood pressure is normal for his age. He continues to vomit even with oral rehydration solution given via a nasogastric tube. Ben's plasma sodium is found to be 156 mmol/L (normal range, 135–145 mmol/L). He needs fluid as he has clinical dehydration. How would this fluid best be replaced?

Select one answer only.

A. Immediate bolus of 20 ml/kg of 0.9% sodium chloride followed by reassessment and replacement of remaining deficit over 24 hours with 0.9% sodium chloride solution
B. Rehydration over 6 hours followed by repeat urea and electrolyte measurement and maintenance fluid only for a further 18 hours
C. Rehydration over 24 hours with 0.18% sodium chloride/5% glucose solution
D. Rehydration over 24 hours with 0.9% sodium chloride/5% glucose solution
E. Rehydration over 48 hours with 0.9% or 0.45% saline

14.8

Matthew is a 3-day-old term infant who has not passed meconium since birth. On examination his abdomen is distended but the remainder of the examination is normal. An x-ray of the abdomen shows distended loops throughout the bowel, including the rectum.

What is the most likely diagnosis?

Select one answer only.

A. Congenital hypothyroidism
B. Cystic fibrosis
C. Duodenal atresia
D. Hirschsprung disease
E. Rectal atresia

Questions: Extended Matching

14.9

The following (A–O) is a list of possible diagnoses which result in vomiting. For each of the following scenarios pick the most likely cause for the vomiting. Each answer may be used once, more than once, or not at all.

A. Appendicitis
B. Coeliac disease
C. Cyclical vomiting syndrome
D. Diabetic ketoacidosis
E. Gastroenteritis
F. Gastro-oesophageal reflux
G. Intussusception
H. Malrotation
I. Meningitis
J. Migraine
K. Pyloric stenosis
L. Raised intracranial pressure
M. Sepsis
N. Strangulated inguinal hernia
O. Urinary tract infection

14.9.1

James, an 8-month-old infant, is bought to the Emergency Department by his parents. He is having episodes of abdominal pain and is just recovering from an upper respiratory tract infection. He seems well in-between, but then suddenly seems to be in pain and looks pale. He has vomited several times. On questioning he has had no blood in his stool but has not opened his bowels for 24 hours.

14.9.2

Bridgitta, an 8-year-old girl, presents to her family doctor with vomiting and abdominal pain. Her vomiting only started today and she has no diarrhoea or fever. She looks unwell and has clinical dehydration on examination and has deep rapid breathing. She is thirsty and pale. She has lost weight over the last few weeks.

14.9.3

Noah is 5 weeks old and has been breastfeeding well and putting on weight. However, over the last 36 hours he has been vomiting after almost every feed. The vomit goes everywhere and he then wants to feed again. All the vomits are milky. He was born at term (birth weight 3.8 kg).

14.9.4

Amir was born by elective caesarean section for maternal pre-eclampsia. His birthweight was 3.3 kg. He is 36 hours old. He has started to establish breastfeeding but has been vomiting after every feed. The vomit is noted by the midwife to be green. On examination his temperature is 37.2°C. His abdomen is slightly distended. The rest of his examination is normal.

14.9.5

Jennifer, a 14-year-old girl, presents to the emergency department with a severe headache for the last 6 hours, mainly affecting the left side of her head. She just wants to lie still in the dark and dislikes being disturbed, but her mother is concerned as she has never had such an episode before and is normally a very lively girl who is doing well at school. She has been vomiting for the last 2 hours and cannot keep anything down and is also complaining of tummy pain. On examination she is distressed by her headache and dislikes having the examination light shone on her. Her temperature is 37.2°C. She does not have neck stiffness or papilloedema. The rest of her examination is normal.

14.10

The following (A–M) is a list of diagnoses associated with abdominal pain in children. For each of the following scenarios select the most likely diagnosis from the list. Each answer may be used once, more than once, or not at all.

A. Appendicitis
B. Coeliac disease
C. Constipation
D. Diabetic ketoacidosis
E. Functional abdominal pain
F. Gastroenteritis
G. Hepatitis
H. Inflammatory bowel disease
I. Inguinal hernia
J. Intussusception
K. Mesenteric adenitis
L. Pneumonia
M. Urinary tract infection

14.10.1

Max, aged 9 years, has been brought to the Emergency Department as he is crying and saying his tummy hurts. He has had a 2-day history of fever and coryza. He has been drinking orange juice but has only eaten some jelly and yogurt. He has not opened his bowels. His temperature is 38.2°C. His throat is red and he has tender cervical lymph nodes. He is not dehydrated. He has mild generalized tenderness of the abdomen, with no guarding.

14.10.2

Pete, aged 4 years, is brought by his mother to the Emergency Department as he is crying and saying his tummy hurts. He has had a 2-day history of fever, coryza and cough. He is sitting quietly on his mother's lap, and is reluctant to play. He has a temperature of 38.2°C and a respiratory rate of 50 beats/min. On examination, his throat is red and he has tender cervical lymph nodes. He complains of tenderness on palpation of the right upper quadrant of the abdomen.

14.10.3

Molly, aged 10 years, is brought to the Paediatric Assessment Unit as she has been vomiting and had central abdominal pain for 2 days. She has also had some diarrhoea. She has only had apple juice and no food for the last day. Her pain is getting worse. On examination, she has a temperature of 38.2°C and a heart rate of 110 beats/min. She has mild dehydration. There is tenderness in the lower right abdomen, but no guarding. When asked to walk, she is unable to stand up straight because of pain.

14.10.4

Francis is 12 years old and is reviewed in the paediatric outpatient department. He has been referred as he has had abdominal pain for the last 3 months. The pain is cramp-like, all over his tummy. He also has developed diarrhoea and is getting up twice in the night to open his bowels. There has not been any blood. He no longer wants to play football in the team, and is increasingly refusing to do his homework. He has lost 1 kg in weight. There are no abnormalities on examination. A blood test shows his haemoglobin level to be 101 g/L, and a raised C-reactive protein of 85 mg/dL (normal <5).

14.10.5

Ted, aged 2 years, has had a 2-day history of low-grade fever and coryza. His mother has brought him to the Emergency Department as he is crying inconsolably. She thinks his tummy is hurting him. He has not opened his bowels for 2 days. He appears reasonably well, has minimal abdominal tenderness but has an indentable mass on the left side of the abdomen.

Answers: Single Best Answer

14.1
A. *Campylobacter*
The most common cause of bloody diarrhoea in the UK. All bacterial forms are notifiable diseases.

B. *Escherichia coli*
This occurs in outbreaks. Verotoxin-producing strains can result in haemolytic uraemic syndrome.

C. *Giardia lamblia*
Giardia lamblia is a parasitic infection and is usually acquired whilst travelling abroad, although there are rare cases in the UK. Persistent diarrhoea would warrant testing for this organism.

D. Rotavirus ⊘
Correct. Rotavirus is a common cause of foul-smelling, watery diarrhoea. *Escherichia coli*, *Shigella*, and *Campylobacter* also cause explosive watery diarrhoea but can be associated with blood in the stools and in the UK are much less common than rotavirus. The incidence of rotavirus in the UK should decline with the introduction of rotavirus vaccine into the standard childhood immunization schedule.

E. *Shigella*
Consider this if there is blood in the stool.

14.2
A. Chronic non-specific diarrhoea
This is not the characteristic history for this condition.

B. Coeliac disease ⊘
Correct. Coeliac disease (gluten-sensitive enteropathy) usually presents at age 8 to 24 months with abnormal stools, faltering growth, abdominal distension, wasting of the muscles of the buttocks (a difficult clinical sign), and irritability. Can also present with short stature or anaemia. It is increasingly detected on screening high-risk groups and at older ages.

C. Hirschsprung disease
Hirschsprung disease presents with constipation and a distended abdomen.

D. Lactose intolerance
Lactose intolerance develops after a bout of gastroenteritis with the child continuing to have diarrhoea. It is usually transient.

E. Ulcerative colitis
Ulcerative colitis usually presents with bloody diarrhoea in older children. Nocturnal waking to defecate associated with abdominal pain should alert you to inflammatory bowel disease.

14.3
A. Chronic non-specific diarrhoea ⊘
Correct. In chronic non-specific diarrhoea there are loose stools with undigested food present. The children grow well and have plenty of energy.

B. Coeliac disease
Although coeliac disease is now relatively common, you would expect more characteristic clinical features. Early weaning (before 3 months) is a risk factor for early onset. Faltering growth is common.

C. Cow's milk protein allergy
Although this is common, affecting at least 1 in 50 children, stools containing undigested food is not characteristic and it is usually accompanied by some atopic markers such as eczema. Parents often report flecks of blood in the stool.

D. Inflammatory bowel disease
Diarrhoea with blood and colicky abdominal pain are characteristic of ulcerative colitis. Crohn's disease usually presents with diarrhoea, abdominal pain and weight loss and general ill health; oral lesions and perianal skin tags are other features.

E. Lactose intolerance
Primary lactose intolerance is common and the norm for many non-Caucasian, non-Arabic populations after infancy. Bloating, discomfort and acidic stool causing perianal soreness are more suggestive. Either a breath test or trial of lactose free diet can be helpful in diagnostic uncertainty. The presence of undigested food in the stool and normal growth are against this diagnosis.

14.4
A. Appendix mass
An appendix mass would be in the right iliac fossa following appendicitis.

B. Constipation ⊘
Correct. The loose stool is overflow from her constipation. Children may present with loose stools when they actually have constipation.

C. Gastroenteritis
Gastroenteritis is unlikely as there is no vomiting and the problem has been going on for a month.

D. Inguinal hernia
An inguinal hernia is not associated with loose stools. It may be associated with pain in the groin or abdomen if it is strangulated, which is not the case in this child. It is also much less common in girls than boys.

E. Wilms tumour
Wilms tumour usually presents as an abdominal mass but as it is a renal mass it would not be confined to the left iliac fossa. Blood in the urine may be present.

14.5

A. Gastro-oesophageal reflux ⊘
Correct. Gastro-oesophageal reflux is caused by the involuntary passage of gastric contents into the lower oesophagus. These infants can vomit several times per day but still continue to gain weight appropriately. If complications are present, it is called gastro-oesophageal reflux disease and needs treatment.

B. *Helicobacter pylori* infection
Helicobacter pylori infection presents with abdominal pain, typically in an older child.

C. Infant colic
Whilst this is common, it is typified by pain (and crying) in the early evening lasting for a few hours. Only a minority of cases are thought to be due to gastro-oesophageal reflux.

D. Overfeeding
Whilst this is a common cause of vomiting, it is uncommon in breastfed babies. The clue in an examination will be that the feed volumes are significantly higher than you would expect. For a bottlefed infant, the feed volume will often be in excess of 200 ml/kg per day.

E. Pyloric stenosis
Although this child has the correct age, there are no 'red flags' to suggest pyloric stenosis. By 8 weeks most affected infants would have either lost weight or at least had a significant plateauing in their weight gain. It is also much less common than reflux. It usually starts to present at a few weeks rather than from birth.

14.6

A. Functional abdominal pain ⊘
Correct. Functional abdominal pain is classically periumbilical and is not associated with any other symptoms. The pain has been going on for 6 months and Claire is well in herself, which suggests that this is not pathological. The pain is very real to her and needs to be explored, as in some children it is a manifestation of stress.

B. Gastritis
Uncommon in this age group and usually felt in the epigastric area when it is the cause. If this was the case, consider testing for *Helicobacter pylori* and if it persists then refer for endoscopy.

C. Hepatitis A
A common infection worldwide but would usually presents with jaundice and dark urine.

D. Irritable bowel syndrome
A diagnosis of exclusion to be made with caution in prepubertal children.

E. Meckel diverticulum
2% of the population have a Meckel diverticulum but in the majority it causes no symptoms. When it does it can be a real diagnostic conundrum but it usually presents with either melaena or fresh blood in the stool. It can also be mistaken for acute appendicitis.

14.7

A. Immediate bolus of 20 ml/kg of 0.9% sodium chloride followed by reassessment and replacement of remaining deficit over 24 hours with 0.9% sodium chloride solution
A bolus of intravenous fluid is not warranted as he is not in shock. Although the pulse rate is not provided, a normal capillary refill time and normal blood pressure confirm this.

B. Rehydration over 6 hours followed by repeat urea and electrolyte measurement and maintenance fluid only for a further 18 hours
As he has hypernatraemic dehydration, rapid rehydration should not be given to avoid potential brain damage from cerebral oedema. This is therefore not a safe plan.

C. Rehydration over 24 hours with 0.18% sodium chloride/5% glucose solution
Rapid rehydration should be avoided to avoid potential brain damage from cerebral oedema. In this case the use of hypotonic sodium chloride solution is dangerous as a rapid fall in serum sodium increases this child's risks. The use of 0.18% sodium chloride solutions is now restricted in the UK.

D. Rehydration over 24 hours with 0.9% sodium chloride/5% glucose solution
In most circumstances rehydration over 24 hours is appropriate; however, in hypernatremic dehydration it is important to make the correction more slowly.

E. Rehydration over 48 hours with 0.9% or 0.45% saline ⊘
Correct. Ben has hypernatremic dehydration, so rehydration must be slow, i.e. over 48 hours to avoid cerebral oedema. In hypernatremic dehydration the brain cells are contracted as water has moved to the extracellular compartment, as this has a higher osmolality (see Fig. 14.1). Changes in extracellular osmolality need to be slow to avoid rapid expansion of cells in the brain.
Hypernatremic dehydration is clinically more difficult to detect than other forms of dehydration on clinical grounds alone (see Fig. 14.1 for reasoning).

14.8

A. Congenital hypothyroidism
Whilst babies with untreated congenital hypothyroidism may develop constipation, it does not cause bowel obstruction.

Hypernatraemic dehydration	Hyponatraemic dehydration
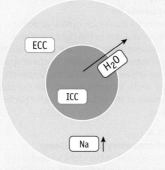	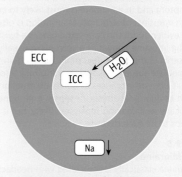
In hypernatraemic dehydration, the sodium concentration in the extracellular compartment (ECC) is increased. Therefore, water moves by osmosis from the intracellular compartment (ICC) to the ECC. So, for a given degree of dehydration, the ECC loses less water than in other types of dehydration. This is why this form of dehydration is readily underestimated clinically.	In hyponatraemic dehydration, the sodium concentration in the ECC is reduced. Therefore, water moves by osmosis from the extracellular to the intracellular compartment. So, for a given degree of dehydration, the ECC loses more volume and the dehydration is readily apparent clinically.

Figure 14.1

B. Cystic fibrosis
Meconium ileus, which is usually a manifestation of cystic fibrosis, causes abdominal distension from bowel obstruction and in some cases a mass may be present. Distension of the colon and rectum would not be a feature.

C. Duodenal atresia
Duodenal atresia causes bile-stained vomiting.

D. Hirschsprung disease ⊘
Correct. Hirschsprung disease is caused by the absence of ganglion cells from the myenteric and submucosal plexuses of part of the large bowel, which results in a narrow, contracted segment. The abnormal bowel extends from the rectum for a variable distance proximally, ending in a normally innervated, dilated colon.

E. Rectal atresia
Rectal atresia causes large bowel obstruction but examination of Matthew's perineum is normal.

Answers: Extended Matching

14.9.1
G. Intussusception
In intussusception there is invagination of one part of the bowel into another. When this occurs, the child cries with pain and goes pale. The passage of redcurrant jelly per rectum from blood-stained mucus is a late sign.

14.9.2
D. Diabetic ketoacidosis
Diabetic ketoacidosis classically presents with a history of weight loss, polydipsia and polyuria. The fast breathing is due to the metabolic acidosis. This can sometimes be mistaken as being a respiratory infection but she is afebrile. A urine dipstick and blood glucose and blood gas will confirm the diagnosis.

14.9.3
K. Pyloric stenosis
This is a typical history. Pyloric stenosis occurs at 2–7 weeks of age; the vomiting is milky and projectile and occurs after each feed. A mass can be felt in the abdomen during or after a test feed. A blood gas will usually show a hypochloremic metabolic alkalosis because chloride and acid are lost from the vomitus. An ultrasound scan of the pylorus is usually diagnostic and is used in many centres to confirm the diagnosis made on clinical examination.

14.9.4
H. Malrotation
Bile-stained vomiting (green vomit) is a red-flag symptom and in a neonate is most likely to be from intestinal obstruction. Malrotation is often not evident until the baby experiences a twisting of the intestine known as a volvulus; it usually presents in the first 3 days of life, and requires immediate surgery. Bilious vomiting may also result from other causes of bowel obstruction, such as duodenal atresia, or sepsis. Amir appears clinically well, making sepsis less likely, but it still needs to be excluded.

14.9.5
J. Migraine
Migraine classically is associated with headache with photophobia and vomiting. It may be accompanied by abdominal pain. Meningitis is a differential diagnosis that should be considered but she is afebrile and does not have any neck stiffness. Cyclical vomiting, by definition, occurs recurrently.

14.10.1
K. Mesenteric adenitis
The mesenteric nodes in the abdomen become inflamed following an upper respiratory tract infection. Can be difficult to differentiate from appendicitis and requires frequent clinical re-assessment to check it resolves. The condition is frequently only diagnosed at laparotomy when a non-inflamed appendix is identified (and removed).

14.10.2
L. Pneumonia
He has tachypnoea, fever and cough. It is important to consider pneumonia as a possible cause of abdominal pain. Laparotomy is not a good treatment for pneumonia!

14.10.3
A. Appendicitis
Appendicitis starts with central abdominal pain that then localizes to the right iliac fossa. Anorexia and loose stools are also associated clinical features. The inability to stand up straight because of pain is known as the 'appendix shuffle' and is adopted to minimize the painful movement of the inflamed adjacent peritoneal surfaces.

14.10.4
H. Inflammatory bowel disease
Getting up during the night to open his bowels is a 'red-flag' sign and should always alert one to the possibility of inflammatory bowel disease. Crohn's disease usually presents with malaise (fever, lethargy, weight loss), which may be accompanied by abdominal pain, diarrhoea, and faltering growth. His anaemia and raised inflammatory markers are consistent with a diagnosis of Crohn's disease.

14.10.5
C. Constipation
Constipation can cause severe abdominal pain and a mass may be palpable on examination. The mass is indentable, which is a sign that this is a faecal mass. The abdomen may be distended but is not tender to touch.

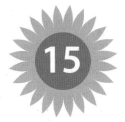

Infection and immunity

Questions: Single Best Answer

15.1

Joseph, aged 3 years, has been unwell for 24 hours with irritability, vomiting and fever. He was seen by his general practitioner earlier in the day and started on amoxicillin. On examination his temperature is 38.5°C, pulse 140 beats/min and blood pressure 90/60 mmHg. He has a rash on his upper limbs and abdomen as shown in Fig. 15.1.

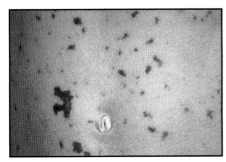

Figure 15.1

What is the most likely diagnosis?

Select one answer only.

A. Henoch–Schönlein purpura
B. Immune thrombocytopenic purpura
C. Measles
D. Meningococcal sepsis
E. Pertussis

15.2

What investigation is most likely to give a definitive diagnosis in Joseph's case?

Select one answer only.

A. Blood culture
B. Lumbar puncture
C. Polymerase chain reaction (PCR)
D. Pernasal swab
E. Throat swab

15.3

Henry is 4 years old and has a 3 day history of fever. He presents to the Accident and Emergency department with a headache. A lumbar puncture is performed. You receive the following result from the laboratory:

- Cerebrospinal fluid (CSF) microscopy:
  - 250 red blood cells/mm^3
  - 1200 neutrophils/mm^3
  - 250 lymphocytes/mm^3
  - CSF protein: 0.6 g/L
  - CSF glucose: 2.1 mmol/L
  - blood glucose: 7.2 mmol/L

What is the most likely diagnosis?

Select one answer only.

A. Bacterial meningitis
B. Blood-stained tap
C. Normal lumbar puncture result
D. Tuberculosis meningitis
E. Viral meningitis

15.4

Graham is 5 years old and has had an intermittent fever for 4 weeks. He presents to the Emergency Department with a headache and neck stiffness. A CT scan is performed, which is normal. A lumbar puncture is performed. You receive the following result from the laboratory:

- cerebrospinal fluid (CSF) microscopy: 95 lymphocytes, 10 neutrophils and 0 red blood cells/mm^3
- CSF protein: 2.2 g/L
- CSF glucose: 1.3 mmol/L
- blood glucose: 6.3 mmol/L

What is the most likely diagnosis?

Select one answer only.

A. Ascending polyneuritis (Guillain–Barré syndrome)
B. Bacterial meningitis
C. Blood-stained tap
D. Tuberculosis meningitis
E. Viral meningitis

15.5

John, a 2-year-old boy, is brought to the general practitioner by his mother. He has the skin rash shown in Fig. 15.2 on both his feet. He also has a few lesions on both hands. They are tender to touch. He is well in himself.

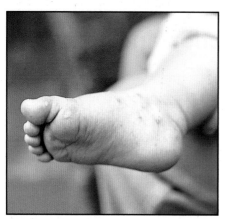

Figure 15.2

What is the most likely cause from the list below?

Select one answer only.

A. Coxsackie A
B. Flea bites
C. Herpes zoster
D. Scabies
E. Varicella zoster

15.6

Ahmed, a 1-year-old boy, is brought to the Paediatric Assessment Unit. He has had a high temperature for the last week. His mother has taken him to the general practitioner on two occasions and he has completed a course of amoxicillin. His eyes are injected and his throat is red. He has marked cervical lymphadenopathy. The skin on his fingers has started to peel. Everyone else in the family is well.

What is the most likely diagnosis?

Select one answer only.

A. Infectious mononucleosis (glandular fever)
B. Kawasaki disease
C. Staphylococcal scalded skin syndrome
D. Scarlet fever
E. Tuberculosis

15.7

Prince, a 4-month-old black African infant, who has recently moved to the UK from Swaziland with his mother is seen in the Paediatric Assessment Unit. He is feeding poorly and is breathless. He has had loose stools for the last 4 weeks and has not put on any weight since then. On examination he appears pale and has marked intercostal recession. His oxygen saturation in air is 82%. His chest X-ray is shown in Fig. 15.3 below.

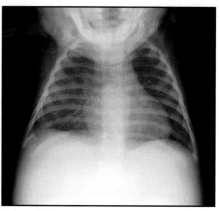

Figure 15.3

What is the most likely cause of his respiratory failure?

Select one answer only.

A. Influenza virus
B. Pneumocystis jiroveci (carinii) pneumonia
C. Respiratory syncytial virus
D. Rhinovirus
E. Staphylococcal pneumonia

15.8

Imran is a 3-year-old boy who moved to the UK from Bangladesh 4 months ago. He has not gained any weight for the last couple of months. He has a cough. The general practitioner has requested a chest X-ray (Fig. 15.4).

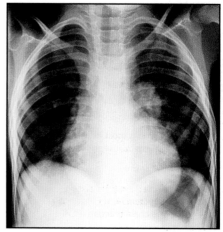

Figure 15.4

What is the most likely diagnosis?

Select one answer only.

A. Asthma
B. Neuroblastoma
C. Pertussis infection
D. Pneumonia
E. Tuberculosis

15.9
You are in the baby clinic at a local general practice. One of the mothers is questioning whether or not she should get her baby immunized as she wonders if it is really necessary. He does not go to nursery and has no siblings so is not at risk of infection.

What advice would you give?

Select one answer only.

A. As most other children are immunized it is not crucial for her child to be immunized as he is unlikely to be exposed to any of the infections in the immunization schedule
B. Immunization is important as a high proportion of children need to be immunized to remove the infections from the community
C. Immunization is important to provide immunity for her child from serious infections and to remove some of these infections from the community
D. It is her choice and you do not feel you should give an opinion
E. Vaccines are associated with side-effects, so you can understand her reasoning

Questions: Extended Matching

15.10
The following (A–T) is a list of infectious agents seen in children. Select the organism that is most likely to be the causative agent in the clinical scenarios outlined below. Each option may be used once, more than once, or not at all.

A. *Aspergillus fumigatus*
B. Chickenpox virus (varicella zoster virus)
C. Cytomegalovirus infection
D. Epstein–Barr virus
E. Herpes simplex virus
F. Human immunodeficiency virus infection
G. Influenza virus
H. Lyme disease (*Borrelia burgdorferi*)
I. Malaria parasites (*Plasmodium* sp.)
J. Measles virus
K. Mumps virus
L. Parvovirus infection (fifth disease)
M. *Pseudomonas aeruginosa*
N. Respiratory syncytial virus
O. Rhinovirus
P. Roseola infantum (sixth disease)
Q. Rubella virus
R. *Staphylococcus aureus*
S. *Streptococcus pneumoniae*
T. Tuberculosis (*Mycobacterium tuberculosis*)

15.10.1
Harry, aged 21 months, presents with a 3 day history of cough and fever and is very miserable and feeding poorly. Examination reveals conjunctivitis and the widespread rash shown in Fig. 15.5 below.

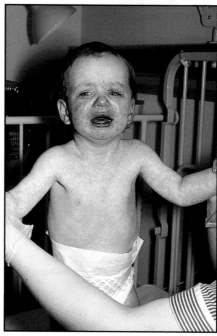

Figure 15.5

15.10.2
Maryam, a 10-month-old infant is brought to her general practitioner. She has had an intermittent fever for 1 day and has a runny nose. Her mother is concerned as her appetite is reduced, but she is still drinking. She is generally miserable when febrile. On examination she has a temperature of 37.9°C, a runny nose and a fine macular rash, mainly on her trunk.

15.10.3
Jennifer, aged 12 years, developed a severe sore throat and lethargy. Amoxicillin was prescribed. The next day she developed the florid maculopapular rash shown (Fig. 15.6).

15.10.4
Sebastian, aged 10 years, has recently returned from a safari holiday in the Kruger National Park in South Africa. He has had a fever for 4 days associated with rigors. Sebastian's blood film is shown in Fig. 15.7 below.

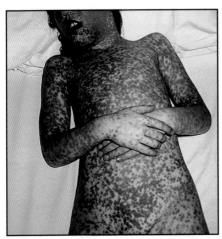

Figure 15.6

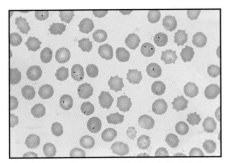

Figure 15.7 (Courtesy of Dr Saad Abdalla).

15.10.5
Philip is 4 years old and has recently started school. He presents with a widespread rash (Fig. 15.8) that is intensely itchy.

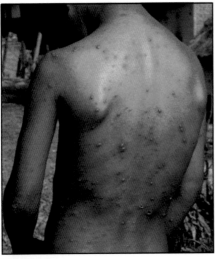

Figure 15.8

15.10.6
Fiona, who is 2 years old, was burnt by a falling mug of tea but it did not seem a bad burn and so her mother did not seek medical attention. The burn developed yellow crusting at the edges and appears to be infected. She now develops profound diarrhoea and collapses. She is admitted to the paediatric intensive care unit. It is noted that she has red lips. She is hypotensive and requires respiratory and circulatory support.

👆 **Hint: Although more than one organism on the list can cause this, the 'yellow crusting' suggests a particular bacterium.**

15.10.7
Katie is 6 years old. She missed a few days of school as she had a fever and was generally lethargic. Now she has a temperature of 38.3°C and has a marked erythematous rash on her cheeks.

👆 **Hint: Also known as 'slapped cheek'.**

15.11
For each of the following patients with an infectious disease, select the NEXT step in management from the list (A–O) below. Each option may be used once, more than once, or not at all.

A. Antipyretic/analgesia
B. Combined anti-tuberculosis medication
C. Highly active antiretroviral therapy
D. Intravenous aciclovir
E. Intravenous antibiotics
F. Intravenous bolus of 20 ml/kg of normal saline
G. Intravenous immunoglobulin
H. Intravenous quinine
I. Nasogastric rehydration therapy
J. Oral antibiotic
K. Oral rehydration solution
L. Oral ACT (artemisinin-based combination therapy)
M. Oxygen
N. Topical antibiotic
O. Topical emollient

15.11.1
Mohammed is 2 years old and presents with a fever and cough for 2 days. He is drinking sips of water but is off his food. He has a temperature of 39.5°C, respiratory rate of 40 breaths/min and his oxygen saturation is normal. On examination he has mild indrawing between his ribs. On auscultation there are some crackles at the left base. There is no wheeze. He is not clinically dehydrated.

15.11.2
Imran is 2 years old and presents with fever and a cough for 2 days. He has a fever of 38°C, a

respiratory rate of 25 breaths/min and oxygen saturation of 98%. He is coryzal and has an inflamed pharynx.

15.11.3
Mustafa, an 18-month-old boy, presents with 3 days of vomiting and diarrhoea. The vomiting has now settled but he continues to have loose stools (he had about eight loose stools in the last 24 hours). His mucous membranes are dry, he has sunken eyes and appears lethargic. His skin turgor is reduced. His extremities are warm and capillary refill time is normal.

15.11.4
Josie is 3 years old. She has had a cough and fever for 6 days. On examination her oxygen saturation is 92% in air. Her temperature is 39°C and she has a respiratory rate of 50 breaths/minute. She has marked indrawing between her ribs and is using her accessory muscles of respiration. On percussion there is 'stony dullness' at her left base and on auscultation decreased air entry at the left base.

15.11.5
Michael is a 2-year-old boy whose parents were born in Taiwan. He has been unwell now for 6 days with a fever, sore eyes and throat. He is noted to have red eyes, an injected throat and cervical lymphadenopathy. He also has a generalized maculopapular rash and the skin is peeling from his hands and feet.

Answers: Single Best Answer

15.1

A. Henoch–Schönlein purpura
Henoch–Schönlein purpura presents with 'palpable' purpura confined to the buttocks and extensor surfaces. It is a clinical diagnosis and often presents with colicky abdominal pain, which may be followed by joint pains.

B. Immune thrombocytopenic purpura
Immune thrombocytopenic purpura often follows a minor viral illness but the child is well; however, the child develops bruising over bony prominences as well as petechiae.

C. Measles
The rash with measles is small reddish brown, flat or slightly raised macules that may coalesce into larger blotchy patches. Usually they first appear on the head or neck, before spreading to the rest of the body.

D. Meningococcal sepsis ⊘
Correct. Meningococcal sepsis is most likely as the child has fever, malaise, and has the characteristic purpuric rash spreading across the abdomen.

E. Pertussis
Whooping cough may cause facial and conjunctival petechiae, but there is no history of cough with this child. Coughing or severe vomiting result in petechiae only in the distribution of the superior vena cava (above the nipples).

15.2

A. Blood culture
Blood culture may be negative as oral bactericidal antibiotics have been given.

B. Lumbar puncture
This would reveal if there was an associated meningitis but a negative result would not rule out septicaemia. The priority in this child is to achieve cardiovascular stability and lumbar puncture should be deferred.

C. Polymerase chain reaction ⊘
Correct. Meningococcal polymerase chain reaction is most likely to give definitive diagnosis. Treatment should not be delayed whilst awaiting results, which may take 2–3 days.

D. Pernasal swab
Pernasal swab is used to diagnose pertussis infection and not meningococcal disease.

E. Throat swab
Throat swab may be negative as oral antibiotics have been given and throat carriage is not indicative of systemic infection.

15.3

A. Bacterial meningitis ⊘
Correct. There is a markedly raised white cell count, mainly neutrophils. The CSF protein is raised, with a reduced ratio of CSF to blood glucose concentration.

B. Blood-stained tap
The red cell count would be much higher if this was to account for the number of white cells present.

C. Normal lumbar puncture result
The CSF results are abnormal. The normal CSF values in a child are:

- white blood cells: 0–5/mm^3
- red blood cells: 0/mm^3
- protein: 0.15–0.4 g/L
- glucose: ≥50% blood glucose.

D. Tuberculosis meningitis
This is rare in the UK and difficult to diagnose. Characteristic findings are lymphocytes rather than neutrophils in the CSF, the CSF protein is markedly raised, and the glucose very low.

E. Viral meningitis
The white blood cells are predominantly lymphocytes rather than neutrophils in the CSF. The neutrophil count may be raised initially in viral meningitis and may predominate in enterovirus infections, but is nearly always less than 1000/mm^3.

15.4

A. Ascending polyneuritis (Guillain–Barré syndrome)
In ascending polyneuritis (Guillain–Barré syndrome), the protein level would also be high but the white cells would not be raised and the glucose would not be so low. It is important to ensure that a paired blood sample is taken for serum glucose.

B. Bacterial meningitis
The white cell count shows predominantly lymphocytes, and the neutrophil count is only marginally raised.

C. Blood-stained tap
No red blood cells are reported in this sample.

D. Tuberculosis meningitis ⊘
Correct. The white cell count shows predominantly lymphocytes. This could also be seen in viral meningitis, but the very markedly raised protein and very low glucose in the CSF together with the clinical history are suggestive of tuberculosis.

E. Viral meningitis
The white cell count shows predominantly lymphocytes. This could also be seen in viral meningitis, but the very markedly raised protein and very low glucose in the CSF together with the clinical history are suggestive of tuberculosis.

15.5

A. Coxsackie A ⊘
Correct. This is hand, foot and mouth disease caused by Coxsackie A. Other infections would not cause painful vesicles in this distribution.

B. Flea bites
These would be itchy. Often other family members would be affected. The soles of the feet would be an unusual site for flea bite marks.

C. Herpes zoster
This would be vesicular and crusting.

D. Scabies
This can be a difficult diagnosis to exclude. Very careful close examination may reveal burrows. Other family members would be likely to have an itchy rash as it is highly contagious.

E. Varicella zoster
This would cause vesicles. They would not be confined to the palms and soles.

15.6

A. Infectious mononucleosis (glandular fever)
Often there are limited signs in this age group although enlarged tonsils with characteristic 'slimy' appearance might prompt testing.

B. Kawasaki disease ⊘
Correct. This is an important diagnosis peculiar to children. He fulfils the major diagnostic criteria of fever for more than 5 days, with cervical lymphadenopathy, injected pharynx, conjunctivitis and peeling fingers. Treatment with intravenous immunoglobulin reduces the risk of coronary artery aneurysm formation.

C. Staphylococcal scalded skin syndrome
There are areas of denuded skin as well as fever and malaise.

D. Scarlet fever
There may be inflammation of the throat but usually a generalized maculopapular rash. This may be followed by peeling of the skin of fingers and toes.

E. Tuberculosis
Failure to respond to antibiotics might make you consider tuberculosis but his clinical features, especially peeling of the skin, do not fit this diagnosis.

15.7

A. Influenza virus
An important cause of fever in the under 1-year-old patient. However, it rarely causes respiratory failure. There would be an adult respiratory distress syndrome pattern on chest X-ray.

B. Pneumocystis jiroveci (carinii) pneumonia ⊘
Correct. This patient is from Swaziland, which markedly increases his risk of HIV infection. All the other infections listed can cause respiratory failure but are less likely in this particular patient. Marked hypoxia in the presence of a relatively normal looking chest X-ray should always make you consider this diagnosis. Prophylactic treatment with cotrimoxazole could have prevented this infection.

C. Respiratory syncytial virus (RSV)
This is the most common cause of bronchiolitis. However, he does not have crepitations and wheeze and his oxygen saturation is much lower than you might expect.

D. Rhinovirus
Some strains of rhinovirus can cause a very severe pneumonitis but they are very rare.

E. Staphylococcal pneumonia
There is no focal consolidation on the chest X-ray as in staphylococcal pneumonia.

15.8

A. Asthma
Asthma can present with a persistent cough, but the X-ray would be normal or the lungs hyperinflated.

B. Neuroblastoma
Malignancy is a possibility, but the chest X-ray and history are suggestive of tuberculosis.

C. Pertussis infection
Pertussis causes a persistent cough, but not these chest X-ray changes.

D. Pneumonia
Bronchopneumonia would make Imran acutely unwell, but there would be consolidation on the chest X-ray.

E. Tuberculosis ⊘
Correct. Tuberculosis is the most likely diagnosis as he has marked left hilar lymphadenopathy on the chest X-ray, and it is endemic in Bangladesh.

15.9

A. As most other children are immunized, it is not crucial for her child to be immunized as he is unlikely to be exposed to any of the infections
This is not true. Herd immunity cannot be guaranteed, as shown by measles outbreaks when immunization rates in the UK dropped following adverse publicity (which was false).

B. Immunization is important, as a high proportion of children need to be immunized to remove the infections from the community
This is true but does not stress the potential benefits to her child and therefore is less likely to be convincing.

C. Immunization is important to provide immunity for her child from serious infections, and to remove some of these infections from the community ⊘
Correct. Immunization would provide benefits to both her child and the wider community.

D. It is her choice, and you do not feel you should give an opinion
Whilst it is her choice to determine whether her child should be immunized, it is important to explore these issues with families to ensure that they are making an informed decision.

E. Vaccines are associated with side-effects, so you can understand her reasoning
However, the risks are much smaller than the potential benefits in every study ever conducted.

Answers: Extended Matching

15.10.1
J. Measles virus
Harry has measles. It is uncommon in countries with immunization programmes, though outbreaks still occur in children who have not been immunized because of parental and public anxiety about the safety of MMR (measles, mumps and rubella) vaccination. It also continues to be a cause of morbidity and death worldwide. Measles virus is a type of paramyxovirus.

15.10.2
O. Rhinovirus
Upper respiratory tract infection is one of the most common problems seen in general practice. The most common causative agent is rhinovirus. This is also the most common trigger for exacerbations of asthma, accounting for more than 80% of exacerbations in children.

15.10.3
D. Epstein–Barr virus
Ampicillin or amoxicillin may cause a florid maculopapular rash in children infected with Epstein–Barr virus (glandular fever) and therefore should be avoided in children who may have glandular fever. If examination reveals 'slimy' enlarged tonsils, this should be suspected.

15.10.4
I. Malaria parasites (*Plasmodium* sp.)
The infection is diagnosed by examination of a thick film. The species (*P. falciparum*, *P. vivax*, *P. ovale*, or *P. malariae*) is confirmed on a thin film. Repeated blood films may be necessary. This blood film shows falciparum malaria.

15.10.5
B. Chickenpox (varicella zoster virus)
Clinical features of chickenpox are fever and itchy, vesicular rash, which crops for up to 7 days.

15.10.6
R. *Staphylococcus aureus*
Fiona has toxic shock syndrome. This is usually caused by a toxin-producing *Staphylococcus aureus*, although group A streptococci can also cause this syndrome. It is characterized by:

- fever ≥39°C
- hypotension
- diffuse erythematous, macular rash
- can also cause mucositis involving conjunctivae, oral and genital mucosa and multiorgan dysfunction.

15.10.7
L. Parvovirus infection (fifth disease)
Parvovirus B19 causes erythema infectiosum or fifth disease, which is also known as 'slapped-cheek syndrome' because of its characteristic facial rash. This infection will temporarily reduce red cell production, which can result in serious anaemia in children with more rapid red cell turnover (hereditary spherocytosis or sickle cell disease) or the fetus.

15.11.1
J. Oral antibiotic
Mohammed has pneumonia. He has cough, fever and focal chest signs. As he does not have an oxygen requirement or signs of a pleural effusion, but has only mild respiratory distress, he can be managed at home with oral antibiotics. The family should be given advice to see a doctor promptly if the breathing becomes more laboured or he becomes more unwell.

15.11.2
A. Antipyretic/analgesia
This child has an upper respiratory tract infection and so can be given an antipyretic/analgesic, i.e. paracetamol. This also has the advantage of making the child more comfortable by easing pain. NICE (National Institute for Health and Care Excellence) guidelines are that fever does not need treating with an antipyretic unless the child is distressed.

15.11.3
K. Oral rehydration solution
This child has gastroenteritis and has clinical dehydration, but is not shocked. This is an important differentiation. As he is not shocked, start with oral rehydration solution, but keep him under observation for about 4 hours to ensure that the oral fluid is tolerated. If not, a nasogastric tube can be sited and fluids given via this route. Intravenous fluids should be avoided where possible.

15.11.4
E. Intravenous antibiotics
Josie has pneumonia with an effusion. She has borderline oxygen saturation and marked respiratory distress and may need oxygen during sleep if her oxygen saturation drops further. Intravenous antibiotics are initially required to treat this infection. When she has been afebrile for 48 hours, this can be changed to oral antibiotics.

15.11.5
G. Intravenous immunoglobulin
Michael has Kawasaki disease and is at risk of developing coronary artery aneurysm, so he requires treatment with intravenous immunoglobulin.

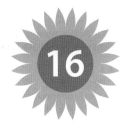
Allergy

Questions: Single Best Answer

16.1

Jonathan, aged 6 years, is brought to the Emergency Department after becoming unwell at a family party. He is unable to say more than a single word and he indicates that he is finding it hard to breathe. He is very anxious. He has a raised itchy rash that is spreading from his face down to his chest. He has never had an episode like this before, although his mother explains that he has asthma and he has been prescribed a salbutamol inhaler previously for wheezy episodes.

What is the most likely diagnosis?

Select one answer only.

A. Acute asthma
B. Allergic reaction
C. Anaphylaxis
D. Idiopathic urticaria
E. Inhaled foreign body

16.2

What will be your first step in Johnathan's management?

Select one answer only.

A. Administer a budesonide nebulizer
B. Assess his airway and give him high-flow oxygen
C. Give intramuscular benzylpenicillin
D. Insert an intravenous cannula
E. Lie him flat

16.3

Cordelia, a 5-month-old infant, was exclusively breastfed up until yesterday when her mother started her on formula as she is planning to go back to work. She noticed that she developed a rash very soon after the formula feed. She has no other medical problems and is not routinely on any medications. On examination she has the rash shown in Fig. 16.1 all over her body.

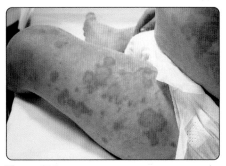

Figure 16.1

What term provides the best description of this rash?

A. Annular
B. Maculopapular
C. Purpuric
D. Urticarial
E. Vesicular

16.4

Eddy is an 8-month-old infant who presents to his general practitioner following a bout of diarrhoea and vomiting, associated with fever for 3 days. This was managed at home with oral rehydration solution. The vomiting had settled but the diarrhoea has continued for three weeks. The stool microscopy and culture were negative. He has no other medical problems and is not on any other medication. On examination he is not dehydrated. He has a soft, mildly distended abdomen.

What is the most likely cause of his prolonged diarrhoea?

A. Coeliac disease
B. Giardiasis
C. IgE mediated cow's milk protein allergy
D. Non-allergic food hypersensitivity
E. Non-IgE mediated cow's milk protein allergy

Answers: Single Best Answer

16.1

A. Acute asthma
The most common reason for admission to hospital in the UK during childhood but the rash points to an allergic cause.

B. Allergic reaction
This is a severe allergic reaction, or anaphylaxis, as it is resulting in difficulty breathing.

C. Anaphylaxis ⊘
Correct. His stridor in association with angioedema and urticaria is characteristic of anaphylaxis. The likely cause is an allergic reaction to a peanut or tree nut encountered at the party.

D. Idiopathic urticaria
This is the most common cause for an urticarial rash but would not account for the sudden onset in difficulty breathing.

E. Inhaled foreign body
This is a common cause of sudden-onset difficulty breathing but would not explain the rash.

16.2

A. Administer a budesonide nebulizer
Nebulized budesonide has been used as a treatment for croup (although it is probably no more effective than oral dexamethasone) but is not the treatment for anaphylaxis.

B. Assess his airway and give him high-flow oxygen ⊘
Correct. Jonathan requires oxygen as he has upper airways obstruction and is having an anaphylactic reaction. Oxygen will improve co-operation and allow time for adrenaline to be drawn up.

C. Give intramuscular benzylpenicillin
This is the treatment for meningococcal septicaemia.

D. Insert an intravenous cannula
The treatment he needs is oxygen and if necessary intramuscular adrenaline.

E. Lie him flat
Lying him flat is contra-indicated as it makes upper airways obstruction worse. If there is no difficulty breathing but signs of shock, then this can be helpful but this is not appropriate in this instance.

16.3

D. Urticarial ⊘
Correct

16.4

A. Coeliac disease
Although this is a possible cause of prolonged diarrhoea, it is less likely than secondary lactose intolerance. If a lactose-free diet does not result in an improvement in symptoms, then this should be considered.

B. Giardiasis
The stool microscopy is negative.

C. IgE mediated cow's milk protein allergy
IgE mediated reactions are rapid and typified by an urticarial reaction.

D. Non-allergic food hypersensitivity ⊘
Correct. This is likely to be temporary lactose intolerance (a non-allergic food hypersensitivity) following gastroenteritis. The stool is likely to have reducing substances in it. This should resolve over several weeks.

E. Non-IgE mediated cow's milk protein allergy
Children with non-IgE mediated cow's milk allergy usually present with faltering growth in conjunction with at least one or more gastrointestinal symptoms including gastroesophageal reflux, loose or frequent stools, abdominal pain, infantile colic, food refusal, constipation and perianal erythema. They are variably affected with atopic eczema.

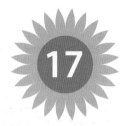

Respiratory disorders

Questions: Single Best Answer

17.1

Liam, a 7-year-old boy, complains to his family doctor of a sore throat and has a mild fever. The appearance of his throat is as shown in Fig. 17.1.

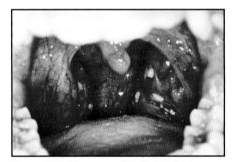

Figure 17.1 (Courtesy of Mr Neil Tolley)

What is the most likely diagnosis?

Select one answer only.

A. Diphtheria
B. Glandular fever (Ebstein Barr virus)
C. Group A Streptococcal tonsillitis
D. Measles
E. Herpes simplex stomatitis

17.2

Mohammed, a 5-year-old refugee from Somalia, presents acutely unwell to the Emergency Department. He has a 1-day history of sore throat and a high temperature (40.1°C). Over the last 8 hours he has been having increasing difficulty breathing with quiet stridor. He has never been immunized. He is noted to be unable to swallow his saliva. Fig. 17.2 was taken when he was intubated.

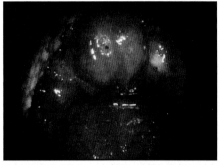

Figure 17.2 (Courtesy of Mr Neil Tolley)

What is the most likely diagnosis?

Select one answer only.

A. Bacterial tracheitis
B. Croup
C. Epiglottitis
D. Foreign body
E. Laryngomalacia

☝ **Hint. When the question stem includes a child who is a refugee the question may be asking indirectly about a disease which is preventable by immunization.**

17.3

Amber, a 9-month-old girl, presents with a 4-day history of coughing spasms which are followed by vomiting. Whooping cough (*Bordetella pertussis* infection) is suspected.

Which of the following tests would be most useful in confirming the diagnosis?

Select one answer only.

A. Blood culture
B. Chest X-ray
C. Full blood count and film
D. Nasopharyngeal aspirate
E. Pernasal swab

17.4

Tak, a 3-year-old Asian boy, presents to his family doctor. He has a 'hacking' cough that started several weeks ago and has failed to respond to two courses of antibiotics. He is otherwise well and has had no previous chest problems. On examination there is decreased air entry in the right lower zone with normal percussion note. His growth is normal.

Which is the most appropriate next step?

Select one answer only.

A. Admit for intravenous antibiotic therapy
B. Assess bronchodilator response
C. Organize for ultrasound-guided drainage of his pleural effusion
D. Request a chest X-ray
E. Request a sweat test and evaluation of immunoglobulins and functional antibodies

17.5

Amir, a 4-year-old boy, presents to his family doctor with a history of eczema, rhinitis, chronic nocturnal cough and intermittent wheeze. Asthma is suspected and a bronchodilator is prescribed.

How should his bronchodilator be delivered?

Select one answer only.

A. Dry powder inhaler
B. Metered dose inhaler (MDI)
C. Metered dose inhaler with large-volume spacer
D. Nebulizer
E. Syrup

17.6

Sarah, a 10-year-old girl, has frequent attacks of asthma. She attends the Emergency Department with increasing difficulty in breathing over the last 12 hours. Initial observation shows that she is anxious, sitting upright, has a marked tracheal tug and is unable to complete a sentence.

Which of the following statements is most likely to be correct?

Select one answer only.

A. Sarah's asthma attack is of moderate severity
B. Sarah's condition is likely to improve if she is encouraged to lie flat
C. Sarah's oxygen saturation should be measured
D. Sarah should be taken promptly to the X-ray department for a chest X-ray
E. The lack of wheeze should make you consider a panic attack

17.7

Zak, a 3-year-old boy, is seen by his general practitioner because of recurrent wheezing associated with upper respiratory tract infections.

Which of the following features most supports the diagnosis of asthma?

Select one answer only.

A. Daytime cough
B. Finger clubbing
C. Peak-flow variability diary
D. Persistent moist cough
E. The presence of symptoms between coughs and colds

17.8

Boris, a 5-month-old infant from Poland, is admitted to hospital with breathing problems and poor feeding. On examination he has a respiratory rate of 50 breaths/min. On auscultation of the chest he has widespread crackles. He has moderate intercostal recession, and oxygen saturation of 92% in air. He was born at term with a birthweight of 3.6 kg (50th centile). His weight is now 5.2 kg (<0.4th centile). This is his first admission to hospital but he 'is always chesty'.

You suspect Boris has cystic fibrosis. When he is stabilized which would be the most appropriate investigation to perform?

Select one answer only.

A. Genetic screening for cystic fibrosis
B. Heel prick for immunoreactive trypsin
C. Measurement of faecal elastase
D. Measurement of serum bilirubin
E. Sweat test

17.9

Norah, an 18-month-old girl, presents to her family doctor with coryza, cough and a mild fever for 3 days. She feeds poorly and is unsettled at night. Her respiratory rate is normal and there is no chest recession.

What is the most likely diagnosis?

A. Bronchiolitis
B. Frontal sinusitis
C. Pneumonia (lower respiratory tract infection)
D. Tonsillitis
E. Upper respiratory tract infection

17.10

Fiona, a 10-month-old infant, has been unsettled and febrile with a runny nose for 2 days. Her family doctor examines her ear canal and the tympanic membrane appears as in Fig. 17.3 below.

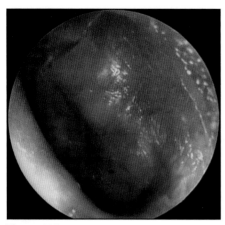

Figure 17.3

What is the most likely diagnosis?

Select one answer only.

A. Acute otitis externa
B. Cholesteatoma
C. Chronic otitis externa
D. Foreign body in the external ear canal
E. Otitis media with effusion

17.11
Jake is a 10-month-old boy from the UK who presents to the Emergency Department with a 2-day history of fever and runny nose. He has been otherwise well. During the night he gradually developed a barking cough in association with a loud noise on inspiration. On examination he has a temperature of 38°C and noisy inspiration accompanied by marked sternal recession (Fig. 17.4). His capillary refill time is normal.

Select the ONE most likely diagnosis from the list below.

A. Acute epiglottitis
B. Anaphylaxis
C. Bronchiolitis
D. Laryngeal foreign body
E. Laryngotracheobronchitis (croup)

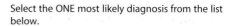

Questions: Extended Matching

17.12
Below is a list of conditions affecting the respiratory tract (A–O). For each of the clinical scenarios described pick the most likely diagnosis from the list. Each answer may be used once, more than once, or not at all.

A. Acute exacerbation of asthma
B. Bronchiolitis obliterans
C. Bronchiolitis
D. Bronchopulmonary dysplasia (BPD)
E. Chronic asthma
F. Cystic fibrosis
G. Inhaled foreign body
H. Laryngotracheobronchitis (croup)
I. Obstructive sleep apnoea
J. Pertussis
K. Pneumonia
L. Pneumothorax
M. Retropharyngeal abscess
N. Tracheitis
O. Tuberculosis

17.12.1
A 10-year-old Caucasian boy has had recurrent chest infections requiring admission to hospital for intravenous antibiotics. He is smaller than his classmates: his weight is on the 2nd centile and height on the 25th centile. His chest X-ray is shown (Fig. 17.5).

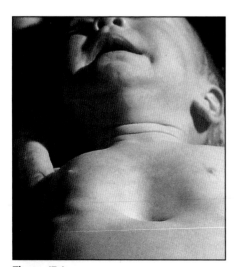

Figure 17.4

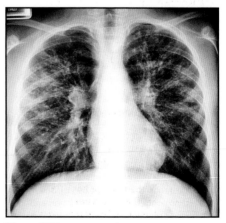

Figure 17.5

17.12.2

A 10-year-old African boy woke up four nights ago with a sudden onset of coughing and choking. Since then he has been noted to be intermittently wheezy. He has wheeze on auscultation of his right chest only. His chest X-ray is shown in Fig. 17.6 below.

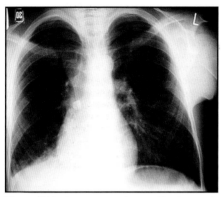

Figure 17.6

17.12.3

A 3-year-old Asian girl has been coughing for 10 days, with fever and lethargy for 2 days. On examination, she has a respiratory rate of 45 breaths/min and crepitations with decreased air entry on her left lung base. Her chest X-ray is shown (Fig. 17.7).

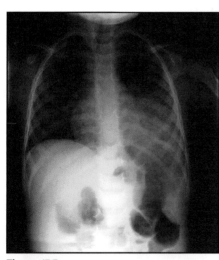

Figure 17.7

17.12.4

Annoushka, a 3-month-old infant, was born at 25 weeks' gestation (birthweight 695 g). She required prolonged artificial ventilation and continues to require oxygen delivered via nasal cannulae. Her chest X-ray is shown (Fig. 17.8).

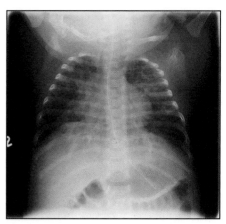

Figure 17.8

17.13

Below is a list of diagnoses (A–N) that result in tachypnoea in children. For each of the following patients with respiratory symptoms, select the most likely diagnosis. Each option may be used once, more than once, or not at all.

A. Acute asthma
B. Bronchitis
C. Bronchiolitis
D. Bronchopulmonary dysplasia (BPD)
E. Chronic asthma
F. Cystic fibrosis
G. Heart failure
H. Inhaled foreign body
I. Laryngotracheobronchitis (croup)
J. Obstructive sleep apnoea
K. Pertussis (whooping cough)
L. Pneumonia
M. Retropharyngeal abscess
N. Tuberculosis

17.13.1

Jamal, a 10-month-old Asian boy, is brought at 1 am to the Emergency Department because he has woken up with noisy breathing. He has had coryzal symptoms for 2 days and now has a barking cough. On examination he has a fever of 37.8°C. He is alert and watches you but clings to his mother. On crying, he has marked inspiratory stridor.

17.13.2

Jack, a 4-month-old infant, has rapid, laboured breathing that has been getting worse over the last 2 days. His mother is concerned as she is struggling to get him to feed. He was born at 27 weeks' gestation, birth weight 979 g and was discharged home at 3 months of age. On examination he has a temperature of 37.4°C and a respiratory rate of 60 breaths/min. He is coughing. His chest is hyperinflated with marked intercostal recession. On auscultation there are generalized fine crackles and wheezes.

17.13.3
Connor, a 5-month-old infant, from a travelling family visiting from Ireland, is admitted to hospital with difficulty breathing and poor feeding. He was born at term with a birthweight of 3.6 kg (50th centile). His weight is now 5.2 kg (<0.4th centile). He has never fed well, and has always tended to regurgitate his milk. This is his first admission to hospital but he 'is always chesty'. On examination he has temperature of 37.9°C, a respiratory rate of 50 breaths/min with widespread crackles on auscultation of the chest.

17.13.4
Fred is a normally well 4-year-old boy. He has had a runny nose and fever for 3 days. He has now developed a cough and difficulty breathing. On examination his temperature is 39°C. He watches you but sits quietly on his mother's lap. He has a respiratory rate of 55 breaths/min. His breaths are rapid but shallow with some mild substernal recession. There is no wheeze on auscultation but some coarse crackles at the right base. His oxygen saturation is 91% in air.

17.13.5
Hannah is a 3-month-old infant who has had a cough for over 2 weeks. She has now developed prolonged bouts of coughing. She has started to vomit at the end of the bout of coughing. Her temperature is 38°C. Her respiratory rate is 25 breaths/min. On auscultation of her chest there are some scattered crackles.

17.14
Below is a list of management options (A–N). For each of the following patients with respiratory disease, select the next step in management. Each option may be used once, more than once, or not at all.

A. Continuous positive airway pressure (CPAP)
B. Endotracheal intubation and ventilation
C. Inhaled salbutamol via metered dose inhaler (MDI)
D. Inhaled salbutamol via MDI and spacer
E. Inhaled steroid via MDI
F. Inhaled steroid via MDI and spacer
G. Intravenous antibiotics
H. Nebulized adrenaline
I. Nebulized salbutamol
J. Nebulized steroid (budesonide)
K. Oxygen therapy
L. Oral antipyretic/analgesic
M. Oral antibiotics
N. Oral corticosteroids

17.14.1
Sara, an 8-month-old Asian girl, presents with a 3-day history of being unsettled. She has been coryzal and has had a mild fever. On examining the right ear canal you note a bulging red tympanic membrane. Her respiratory rate is 25 breaths/min and she does not have any chest recession.

17.14.2
Chardonnay is a 6-year-old Caucasian girl who has asthma. Her mother smokes cigarettes and there is poor compliance with her preventative steroid therapy. She presents with a 2-day history of cough, runny nose, mild fever and 'breathlessness'. Her mother cannot remember her previous peak-flow result. On examination she has a respiratory rate of 30 breaths/min, mild intercostal recession and oxygen saturation of 96% in air.

17.14.3
Jake, a 7-month-old infant, presents with a 2-day history of fever and runny nose. During the night he has developed a harsh cough in association with noisy inspiration. On examination, you note he has moderate stridor mainly on inspiration and mild intercostal and subcostal recession. His respiratory rate is 30 breaths/min. He has a temperature of 37.8°C. His capillary refill time is normal. His oxygen saturation is 96% in air.

Answers: Single Best Answer

17.1

A. Diphtheria
Diptheria is now extremely rare as children are immunized in the UK. Also the appearance is not 'typical'. In diphtheria a thick grey pharyngeal membrane is characteristic.

B. Glandular fever (Ebstein Barr virus)
Infection with Ebstein Barr virus can lead to tonsillitis although typically the tonsils are coated with a grey membrane. Palatal petechiae (pinpoint spots on the soft palate) may also be seen.

C. Group A Streptococcal tonsillitis ⊘
Correct. There is intense inflammation of the tonsils with purulent exudates. In this age group Group A beta-haemolytic *Streptococcus* is the most likely causative pathogen.

D. Measles
In measles there may be white spots (Koplik spots) visible on the buccal mucosa.

E. Herpes simplex stomatitis
There are lesions on the lips, gums and tongue.

17.2

A. Bacterial tracheitis
The child would have loud, harsh stridor and would not have an enlarged epiglottis as shown in the figure.

B. Croup
The child would be less seriously unwell or 'toxic' and would have a mild fever and loud stridor and would not have the abnormal appearance shown in the figure.

C. Epiglottitis ⊘
Correct. The photograph shows the characteristic grossly enlarged 'cherry red' epiglottis of acute epiglottitis. It is caused by *Haemophilus influenzae* type b. In the UK and many other countries, the introduction of universal *H. influenzae* type b immunization in infancy has led to a >99% reduction in the incidence of epiglottitis and other invasive *H. influenzae* type b infections.

D. Foreign body
The history would be of a sudden onset of cough or respiratory distress, and there would not be a high fever.

E. Laryngomalacia
The child would not be unwell and would have had recurrent or continuous stridor since infancy. Laryngomalacia generally resolves within the 1st year of life.

17.3

A. Blood culture
It is incredibly rare to isolate *Bordetella pertussis* from blood cultures.

B. Chest X-ray
Chest X-ray changes can occur in whooping cough but are not diagnostic.

C. Full blood count and film
A marked lymphocytosis is characteristic of pertussis, but not diagnostic. The lymphocytosis is secondary to pertussis toxin. *Bordetella parapertussis* does not produce pertussis toxin.

D. Nasopharyngeal aspirate
Immunofluorescence of a nasopharyngeal aspirate is used to identify respiratory syncytial virus, which causes bronchiolitis, but is not helpful in the diagnosis of pertussis.

E. Pernasal swab ⊘
Correct. Culturing a pernasal swab allows the pathogen (*Bordetella pertussis*) to be identified (though PCR (polymerase chain reaction) is more sensitive). This can also be helpful in isolating the related *Bordetella parapertussis*.

17.4

A. Admit for intravenous antibiotic therapy
Tak has already failed to respond to two courses of antibiotics, so further investigation is warranted.

B. Assess bronchodilator response
There is no wheeze on examination and so inhaled bronchodilator is unlikely to be effective.

C. Organize for ultrasound-guided drainage of his pleural effusion
His signs are not consistent with a pleural effusion. The percussion note would be stony dull if this was a pleural effusion.

D. Request a chest X-ray
The most likely diagnosis is the inhalation of a foreign body, e.g. a peanut. Tak also has focal chest signs and so needs a chest X-ray to be performed.

E. Request a sweat test and evaluation of immunoglobulins and functional antibodies
A sweat test is used to diagnose cystic fibrosis and is not indicated here because this is his first episode of chest problems and he is growing normally. Functional antibodies and immunoglobulins are useful screening tests for possible immunodeficiency and this 'triad' of investigations is often used in children with faltering growth and/or recurrent respiratory infections.

17.5

A. Dry powder inhaler
Dry powder inhaler is appropriate only if MDI and spacer have failed in this age group. Most 4 year olds will perform better with MDI and spacer.

B. Metered dose inhaler (MDI)
Children should be prescribed a MDI with spacer as they cannot co-ordinate an MDI alone. It is always preferable to use a spacer, even in adults as delivery is more reliable.

C. Metered dose inhaler with large-volume spacer ⊘
Correct. The best mode of delivery is direct to the lungs. Children under 5 years of age should be prescribed a MDI with spacer as they cannot co-ordinate an MDI alone.

D. Nebulizer
Nebulizers provide very effective delivery of bronchodilators. However, they produce more hypoxia than bronchodilators delivered by pressurized MDI and spacer, are more expensive, and are not as safe. In hospital the nebulizers are driven by oxygen to offset the risk.

E. Syrup
Syrup should not be used as it is results in high blood levels and unacceptable side-effects.

17.6

A. Sarah's asthma attack is of moderate severity
Sarah's attack is severe as she is unable to complete a sentence.

B. Sarah's condition is likely to improve if she is encouraged to lie flat
Sitting upright assists lung mechanics and enables her to use her accessory muscles.

C. Sarah's oxygen saturation should be measured ⊘
Correct. Oxygen saturation should be measured to further assess the severity of the asthma attack and to guide treatment.

D. Sarah should be taken promptly to the X-ray department for a chest X-ray
The priority is to treat Sarah's asthma. If a chest X-ray is indicated, then a portable X-ray machine should be brought to any patient who is significantly unwell.

E. The lack of wheeze should make you consider a panic attack
The absence of wheeze implies that little air is moving in and out of the chest and would indicate severe bronchoconstriction.

17.7

A. Daytime cough
Nocturnal cough is classically experienced with asthma. A cough that always resolves during sleep is likely to be habitual (psychogenic).

B. Finger clubbing
Clubbing suggests suppurative lung disease or congenital heart disease.

C. Peak-flow variability diary
Zak is too young to perform peak flow reliably.

D. Persistent moist cough
This suggests persistent bacterial bronchitis.

E. The presence of symptoms between coughs and colds ⊘
Correct. The presence of interval symptoms and atopic conditions (eczema/hay fever) helps to distinguish asthma from viral-induced wheeze.

17.8

A. Genetic screening for cystic fibrosis
ΔF508 is the most common mutation in cystic fibrosis, but is not diagnostic as some children with cystic fibrosis will have a different mutation. Even screening for the most common mutations will miss some affected children. If the sweat test is positive or borderline, then genetic screening is helpful in determining prognosis. Some mutations are associated with milder disease or may be amenable to treatment.

B. Heel prick for immunoreactive trypsin
Immunoreactive trypsin remains high (elevated) only for a few weeks before returning to normal levels. This test is used for newborn screening.

C. Measurement of faecal elastase
Children with untreated cystic fibrosis will have low faecal elastase and faltering weight. This confirms pancreatic insufficiency. However, cystic fibrosis is not the only cause for this and a sweat test will still be required.

D. Measurement of serum bilirubin
Cystic fibrosis can cause prolonged jaundice (>14 days of age), but this is not specific.

E. Sweat test ⊘
Correct. Abnormal function of the sweat glands results in excessive concentrations of sodium and chloride in the sweat, and this is the basis of the essential diagnostic test for cystic fibrosis.

17.9

A. Bronchiolitis
Norah's chest has no abnormal signs on auscultation. With bronchiolitis, you would expect to hear crepitations and wheeze, and to see signs of respiratory distress.

B. Frontal sinusitis
This is unusual in children of this age because frontal sinuses do not develop until late childhood.

C. Pneumonia (lower respiratory tract infection)
Young children with pneumonia can sometimes present without chest signs on auscultation, but

there would be respiratory distress including a raised respiratory rate.

D. Tonsillitis
Examination of the oropharynx would show intense inflammation of the tonsils, often with a purulent exudate.

E. Upper respiratory tract infection ✓
Correct. This child has an upper respiratory tract infection, most likely a common cold.

17.10
A. Acute otitis externa
Acute otitis externa is an infection of the outer ear canal, not of the tympanic membrane.

B. Cholesteatoma
A rare problem in children. The two most common symptoms are persistent, often smelly, discharge from the affected ear and gradual loss of hearing in the affected ear.

C. Chronic otitis externa
Chronic otitis externa is an infection of the outer ear canal, not of the tympanic membrane. Fiona's history is only 2 days long and therefore not chronic.

D. Foreign body in the external ear canal
Fiona has symptoms of an upper respiratory tract infection and fever, and no foreign body is seen on examination.

E. Otitis media with effusion ✓
Correct. Here the ear drum is dull and bulging.

17.11
A. Acute epiglottitis
Epiglottitis would present with a shorter history, and the child would be extremely unwell (toxic). It is also very rare in the UK and countries with *Haemophilus influenzae* type b immunization.

B. Anaphylaxis
Anaphylaxis may cause stridor but also causes other symptoms, often including an urticarial rash. It would not cause a fever.

C. Bronchiolitis
Bronchiolitis causes wheeze and crepitations rather than stridor as in this child.

D. Laryngeal foreign body
The child has a fever and a gradual onset of symptoms.

E. Laryngotracheobronchitis (croup) ✓
Correct. Laryngotracheobronchitis (croup) is mucosal inflammation and increased secretions affecting the airway. Croup occurs from 6 months to 6 years of age. Fever suggests infection. Inspiratory noises suggest upper airway obstruction.

Answers: Extended Matching

Answer 17.12.1
F. Cystic fibrosis
The history of recurrent severe chest infections with poor weight gain is suggestive of cystic fibrosis. The chest X-ray shows extensive changes with large-volume lungs with extensive reticulonodular shadowing, and peribronchial thickening with hilar lymphadenopathy, consistent with cystic fibrosis. With screening, late presentation like this will become uncommon.

Answer 17.12.2
G. Inhaled foreign body
The acute history of coughing and focal wheeze is suggestive of an inhaled foreign body. The tooth is visible in the right main bronchus.

Answer 17.12.3
K. Pneumonia
The history of fever, cough and being unwell (lethargy), with signs of tachypnoea and focal crepitations are suggestive of pneumonia. The chest X-ray shows that there is loss of contour of the left heart border and of the left hemidiaphragm.

Answer 17.12.4
D. Bronchopulmonary dysplasia (BPD)
Preterm infants who still have an oxygen requirement at a postmenstrual age of 36 weeks are described as having bronchopulmonary dysplasia (BPD). The lung damage may be caused by pressure and volume trauma from artificial ventilation, oxygen toxicity and infection, but delay in lung maturation is now the most common predisposing factor. The chest X-ray, as shown here, characteristically shows widespread areas of opacification, sometimes with cystic changes.

Answer 17.13.1
I. Laryngotracheobronchitis (croup)
Jamal has laryngotracheobronchitis (croup). This is the correct diagnosis because he has stridor accompanied by a low-grade fever, a viral upper respiratory tract infection, and is alert.

Answer 17.13.2
C. Bronchiolitis
Jack has signs and symptoms of bronchiolitis, including poor feeding, increased work of breathing, mild fever, cough and crackles and wheeze on auscultation. Jack is at increased risk of respiratory failure from bronchiolitis because he was preterm.

Answer 17.13.3
F. Cystic fibrosis
The clinical features suggesting cystic fibrosis are respiratory infection together with being 'always chesty' and poor weight gain since birth and his

Irish descent (the cystic fibrosis gene frequency is particularly high in Ireland). Routine screening is performed on the newborn biochemical blood test at about 5 days of age. However, he may have missed the screening because the test is done at home following discharge from hospital and he is from a travelling community.

Answer 17.13.4
L. Pneumonia
Fred has signs and symptoms of pneumonia, including tachypnoea, fever, and localized crepitations, as well as a preceding viral upper respiratory tract infection.

Answer 17.13.5
K. Pertussis (whooping cough)
This infant has paroxysms of coughing, which are so severe that they cause her to vomit. This is suggestive of pertussis. The characteristic inspiratory whoop may be absent in infants, but apnoea can be a feature at this age. Vaccination reduces the risk of developing pertussis and reduces the severity of disease in affected infants but does not guarantee protection. Maternal immunization against pertussis should reduce the risk of their infants developing the disease.

Answer 17.14.1
L. Oral antipyretic/analgesic
This child has acute otitis media. Pain should be treated with an analgesic such as paracetamol.

Around 80% of cases of acute otitis media resolve spontaneously. Antibiotics marginally shorten the duration of pain but have not been shown to reduce the risk of hearing loss, and there is an increased risk of minor side-effects. They would be indicated if the child is still unwell after 48 hours.

Answer 17.14.2
D. Inhaled salbutamol via metered dose inhaler and spacer
Chardonnay has an acute exacerbation of asthma of moderate severity. She should be given a high dose of bronchodilator via a metered dose inhaler and spacer. Using a nebulizer is no more effective (and might encourage her mother to attend hospital again as she does not have one at home). She does not need oxygen as her oxygen saturation is normal in air.

Answer 17.14.3
N. Oral corticosteroid
Jake has croup of moderate severity. Nebulized steroid (budesonide) or oral corticosteroids have been shown to reduce the severity of croup and need for hospitalization. However, nebulizers are more costly and have no advantage over oral corticosteroids. In the UK oral dexamethasone rather than prednisolone is usually used as it has a longer half-life.

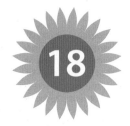

Cardiac disorders

Questions: Single Best Answer

18.1
Alan, a 4-month-old boy, sees his general practitioner for an ear infection. On listening to his chest a heart murmur is heard.

Which one of the following features most suggests that it requires further investigation?

Select one answer only.

A. A thrill
B. Disappearance of murmur on lying flat
C. Murmur maximal at the left sternal edge
D. Sinus arrhythmia
E. Systolic murmur

18.2
Which of the following is the most common type of congenital heart disease in the UK?

Select one answer only.

A. Atrial septal defect
B. Persistent arterial duct
C. Pulmonary stenosis
D. Tetralogy of Fallot
E. Ventricular septal defect

18.3
Sunil, a 3-month-old infant, presents with breathlessness and sweating on feeding. He has had several chest infections. You suspect heart failure.

Which of the following is most likely to be correct regarding his heart failure?

Select one answer only.

A. Hepatomegaly is not a common feature at this age
B. It is caused by Eisenmenger syndrome
C. It is due to left heart obstruction
D. It is due to a left-to-right shunt
E. It is due to an increase in right-to-left shunt

18.4
Tariq, who is 6 weeks old, is admitted directly from the cardiology clinic with heart failure. He has a large ventricular septal defect. The cardiologist has recommended treatment with furosemide and spironolactone. His mother wants to know why he has only now started to have problems. Which of the following statements provides the best explanation?

Select one answer only.

A. At birth and for the first few weeks the ductus arteriosus remained patent and this balanced the flow across the septal defect
B. Pulmonary vascular resistance is increasing and blood is now flowing from right to left
C. The left ventricle is now failing due to its progressive dilatation
D. The pulmonary vascular resistance falls after birth and now flow from left to right across the septal defect is much greater
E. Volume overload results in decreased return to the left ventricle and a reduction in cardiac output related to a reduced end-diastolic filling pressure

18.5
John, who is 6 years old, presents to the Emergency Department feeling sick and dizzy. He was brought to hospital by a paramedic crew who were called after he became unwell at school. His heart rate was noted to be very quick, at 260 beats/min and supraventricular tachycardia is diagnosed. He says he can feel his heart beating quickly and looks pale. He is crying, saying he wants his mother.

Which of the following should be undertaken by the attending team?

Select one answer only.

A. Adenosine via a large bore intravenous line
B. Bilateral carotid sinus massage
C. Direct current cardioversion
D. Reassure that it will resolve spontaneously
E. Vagal stimulation manoeuvre

Questions: Extended Matching

18.6
The following is a list (A–J) of congenital heart problems encountered in children. From the list select the most likely diagnosis given the associated findings on clinical examination.

A. Aortic stenosis
B. Atrial septal defect
C. Coarctation of the aorta
D. Dextrocardia
E. Mitral regurgitation
F. Mitral stenosis
G. Normal
H. Persistent ductus arteriosus
I. Ventricular septal defect
J. Pulmonary stenosis

The site and heart sounds and murmurs are depicted below in Fig. 18.1. For each presentation, select the most likely diagnosis.

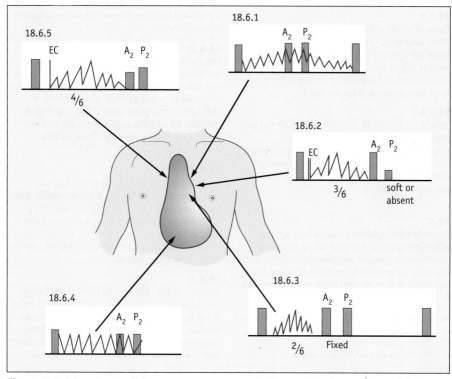

Figure 18.1. EC = ejection click. A2 = aortic component of second heart sound. P2 = pulmonary component of second heart sound.

18.7
Below is a list (A–M) of possible findings on echocardiography. For each of the following clinical scenarios described select the most likely findings on echocardiography. Each option may be used once, more than once, or not at all.

A. Aortic stenosis
B. Atrial septal defect
C. Coarctation of the aorta
D. Dextrocardia with situs inversus
E. Dextrocardia with situs solitus
F. Mitral regurgitation
G. Mitral stenosis
H. Normal
I. Persistent ductus arteriosus
J. Pulmonary stenosis
K. Tetralogy of Fallot
L. Transposition of the great arteries
M. Ventricular septal defect

18.7.1
Jack is 24 hours old and his mother notices when he is about to breastfeed that he is blue around the mouth. On examination, his tongue looks blue and there is peripheral cyanosis. His respiratory rate is 65 breaths/min. On auscultation of the chest there is no murmur. Pulses in all four limbs can be palpated and are equal in volume. He is watching you and moving his arms and legs vigorously whilst you examine him.

18.7.2

Sarah was born at term by spontaneous vaginal delivery and went home at 8 hours of age following a normal neonatal discharge examination. At 48 hours of age her mother found her looking pale and was unable to wake her. She was rushed to the Emergency Department. Her breathing was noted to be very shallow, her skin was cool and mottled and she was unresponsive to pain. She is resuscitated, and given intravenous fluids and broad-spectrum antibiotics. On examination, the only palpable pulse is the right brachial pulse.

18.7.3

Azam, a 5-year-old boy, presents with frequent chest infections. On examination of the chest there are bilateral crackles at the bases. His heart sounds can be heard throughout the praecordium but are louder on the right. His apex beat is palpable on the right.

18.7.4

Jane, a previously fit and well 18-month-old girl, presents with frequent respiratory tract infections and wheeze. On examination there is a fixed and widely split second heart sound, an ejection systolic murmur best heard at the upper left sternal edge.

18.8

Below is a list (A–M) of possible findings on echocardiography. For each of the following children who present with a heart murmur select the most likely findings on echocardiography. Each option may be used once, more than once, or not at all.

A. Aortic stenosis
B. Atrial septal defect
C. Coarctation of the aorta
D. Dextrocardia with situs inversus
E. Dextrocardia with situs solitus
F. Mitral regurgitation
G. Mitral stenosis
H. Normal
I. Persistent ductus arteriosus
J. Pulmonary stenosis
K. Tetralogy of Fallot
L. Transposition of the great arteries
M. Ventricular septal defect (VSD)

18.8.1

Anoushka, a 1-year-old girl, presents to the Emergency Department with a respiratory tract infection. She is pink and well-perfused. There is a thrill and pansystolic murmur at the lower left sternal edge.

18.8.2

Debbie, a 3-month-old female infant is being reviewed in the paediatric outpatient clinic. She was referred as on her 6-week check the general practitioner heard a continuous murmur throughout the praecordium. She is well and thriving. All peripheral pulses are present and easily palpable. Oxygen saturation is 96% post-ductal.

18.8.3

Nada, a 5 month old female infant has a fever and runny nose for 2 days. On examination she has a fever of 38.3°C and a runny nose. Her tongue is pink. Her breathing is normal. Pulse is 160 beats/min. Her heart sounds are normal but she has a soft systolic murmur at the left sternal edge. Pulses are normal.

18.8.4

Robert, a 3-year-old boy, has had a runny nose and wheeze for 3 days. On examination his pulse is 100 beats/min. Pulses are normal. There is an ejection systolic murmur heard loudest at the upper right sternal edge, which can also be heard over the carotid arteries but not at the back.

Answers: Single Best Answer

18.1

A. A thrill ✓
Correct. A thrill is a palpable murmur, i.e. a loud murmur. It always requires further investigation.

B. Disappearance of murmur on lying flat
The disappearance of the murmur on lying flat is characteristic of a venous hum, which is innocent.

C. Murmur maximal at the left sternal edge
Murmurs at the left sternal edge may be innocent or pathological. Further investigation is not indicated if the features of an innocent murmur are fulfilled.

D. Sinus arrhythmia
Sinus arrhythmia is a variation in heart rate with respiration and is a normal finding in children.

E. Systolic
Systolic murmurs may be innocent or pathological. Hallmarks of an innocent ejection murmur (all have an 'S', therefore innoSent) are:
- aSymptomatic patient
- soft blowing murmur
- systolic murmur only, not diastolic
- left sternal edge.

Additional requirements are:
- normal heart sounds with no added sounds
- no parasternal thrill
- no radiation.

Further investigation is not indicated under these circumstances.

18.2

E. Ventricular septal defect ✓
Correct. This is the most common single group of structural congenital heart disease (30%).

18.3

A. Hepatomegaly is not a common feature at this age
Hepatomegaly is an important clinical feature of heart failure in children at all ages. Percussion of the upper border of the liver will help discriminate between hepatomegaly and downward displacement of a liver from hyperexpansion of the chest.

B. It is caused by Eisenmenger syndrome
Eisenmenger syndrome causes cyanosis from pulmonary hypertension, and usually occurs in the second decade of life.

C. It is due to left heart obstruction
Only in the 1st week of life is heart failure usually from left heart obstruction, e.g. coarctation of the aorta.

D. It is due to a left-to-right shunt ✓
Correct. After the 1st week of life, progressive heart failure is most likely due to a left-to-right shunt, most often from a ventricular septal defect.

E. It is due to an increase in right-to-left shunt
It is due to increasing left-to-right shunt.

18.4

A. At birth and for the first few weeks the ductus arteriosus remained patent and this balanced the flow across the septal defect
A ventricular septal defect is not a 'duct-dependent' lesion. A widely open ductus will not prevent heart failure here.

B. Pulmonary vascular resistance is increasing and blood is now flowing from right to left
This is Eisenmenger syndrome and would not occur in a 6-week-old baby. It is a late complication of untreated ventricular septal defect/atrioventricular septal defect.

C. The left ventricle is now failing due to progressive dilation
Dilated cardiomyopathy is a very late change. In children with ventricular septal defect the heart remains healthy but heart failure occurs from volume overload.

D. The pulmonary vascular resistance falls after birth and now flow from left to right across the septal defect is much greater ✓
Correct. The pulmonary vascular resistance falls over the first few weeks of life. This increases the flow across the septal defect and leads to progressively worsening heart failure.

E. Volume overload results in decreased return to the left ventricle and a reduction in cardiac output related to a reduced end-diastolic filling pressure
In hypovolemic shock there is decreased cardiac filling leading to heart failure. However, this is the result of hypovolemia rather than volume overload and is not the case here.

18.5

A. Adenosine via a large bore intravenous line
This is likely to be effective but should be tried only after vagal manoeuvres have been undertaken.

B. Bilateral carotid sinus massage
Whilst this might work, it should not be undertaken bilaterally as this might be dangerous.

C. Direct current cardioversion
This is painful and even synchronized shock requires a general anaesthetic first.

D. Reassure that it will resolve spontaneously
He is symptomatic and it should be treated.

E. Vagal stimulation manoeuvre ✓
Correct. Instruct John how to perform a Valsalva manoeuvre – ask him to put his thumb in his mouth and try to blow on it like a trumpet; this often works. Cold ice pack to the face is an alternative.

Answers: Extended Matching

Answer 18.6.1
H. Persistent ductus arteriosus
There is flow during systole and diastole suggesting that there is a pressure gradient in both. This makes one think of a shunt between arteries – in this case the aorta to the pulmonary artery across the persistent ductus arteriosus.

Answer 18.6.2
J. Pulmonary stenosis
An ejection click tells you this is a valvular problem. The quiet P2 suggests the pulmonary valve is the source. A difficult set of signs to detect clinically.

Answer 18.6.3
B. Atrial septal defect.
The variation in timing of closure of aortic and pulmonary valves is lost when there is an atrial septal defect. The fixed and widely split second heart sound (often difficult to hear) is due to the right ventricular stroke volume being equal in both inspiration and expiration.

Answer 18.6.4
I. Ventricular septal defect
The lack of an opening click and the presence of a pansystolic murmur are highly suggestive of ventricular septal defect. In general, all pansystolic murmurs are appreciated most easily below the level of the nipples.

Answer 18.6.5
A. Aortic stenosis
An ejection click tells one this is a valvular problem. The quiet A2 suggests that the aortic valve is the source. A difficult set of signs to detect clinically. In clinical practice radiation to the neck (or a suprasternal thrill) is a useful sign of left outflow tract obstruction.

Answer 18.7.1
L. Transposition of the great arteries
He has cyanotic congenital heart disease. This is transposition of the great arteries as all his pulses are present on examination. This is also classically the age when this presents.

Answer 18.7.2
C. Coarctation of the aorta
Collapse of a newborn can be caused by: septicaemia/meningitis, congenital heart disease or an inborn error of metabolism. In this case the likely diagnosis is outflow obstruction in a sick neonate – severe coarctation of the aorta or interrupted aortic arch. When the ductus arteriosus closes, perfusion of the left arm and lower body is compromised. Performing a four-limb blood pressure measurement might help confirm the diagnosis, with the blood pressure in the legs being lower than in the right arm.

Answer 18.7.3
D. Dextrocardia with situs inversus
The right-sided apex indicates dextrocardia. This may be associated with primary ciliary dyskinesia (Kartagener syndrome), which is likely to be responsible for his frequent respiratory infections. Cilia are required to decide the polarity of an embryo. Without adequate ciliary function, the lateralization of organs occurs randomly and therefore approximately half of children will have dextrocardia with situs inversus (stomach on the right and liver on the left). Isolated dextrocardia with situs solitus (with the stomach and liver in their normal positions) is not a ciliary problem.

Answer 18.7.4
B. Atrial septal defect
An atrial septal defect. This classically presents with an ejection systolic murmur best heard at the upper left sternal edge – due to increased flow across the pulmonary valve because of the left-to-right shunt. The fixed and widely split second heart sound (often difficult to hear) is due to the right ventricular stroke volume being equal in both inspiration and expiration.

Answer 18.8.1
M. Ventricular septal defect
Children with VSDs may have recurrent chest infections. VSDs classically present with a pansystolic murmur loudest at the left sternal edge.

Answer 18.8.2
I. Persistent ductus arteriosus
Most children present with a continuous murmur beneath the left clavicle. The murmur continues into diastole because the pressure in the pulmonary artery is lower than that in the aorta throughout the cardiac cycle. Some sources describe the murmur as sounding like 'machinery'. Whilst it varies in intensity during the cardiac cycle (it is usually loudest in systole and quieter but still present in diastole), the key feature is its presence throughout systole and diastole. The pulse pressure is increased, causing collapsing or bounding pulses, making them easy to feel.

Answer 18.8.3
H. Normal
Innocent murmurs can often be heard in children. It is obviously important to be able to distinguish an innocent murmur from a pathological one. During a febrile illness or anaemia, innocent or flow murmurs are often heard because of increased cardiac output.

Answer 18.8.4

A. Aortic stenosis

It can be difficult to discriminate between left and right outflow tract obstruction as both result in ejection systolic murmurs. Opening clicks indicate valvular involvement but they are difficult to hear even with experience. The presence of radiation to the neck and/or a suprasternal thrill is a very useful sign and is a feature of left-sided obstruction.

Kidney and urinary tract disorders

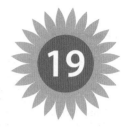

Questions: Single Best Answer

19.1

Emily is a 2-year-old girl. She presents to the Emergency Department with a 2-day history of fever, vomiting and 'smelly' urine. She has no significant medical history and is not on any medication. On examination she has a temperature of 39°C and has a heart rate of 126 beats/min. She has generalized tenderness over her abdomen.

What is the best way to collect a urine sample from her?

Select one answer only.

A. Bag sample
B. Catheter sample
C. Clean catch
D. Pad/cotton wool balls in nappy
E. Suprapubic aspirate

19.2

Becky is a 7-year-old girl. She is seen by her general practitioner with a 2-day history of fever and abdominal pain. Her mother has noted that she is going to the toilet to pass urine more often than usual. On examination she is now afebrile and has no abdominal tenderness.

What is the most likely diagnosis?

Select one answer only.

A. Appendicitis
B. Cystitis
C. Diabetic ketoacidosis
D. Glomerulonephritis
E. Pyelonephritis

19.3

Jonathan is an 8-year-old boy. He has a medical history of urinary tract infections. On this occasion he presents to hospital with acute spasmodic pain on the left side of his abdomen. He says it is the worst pain he has ever experienced. He played football yesterday but had not hurt himself. On examination he is afebrile and his abdomen is soft with no guarding. He is tender in his left loin and there are no palpable masses. He has 2+ of haematuria on dipstick of his urine but no protein or leucocytes. He is not on any medication.

What is the most likely cause of his pain?

Select one answer only.

A. Constipation
B. Glomerulonephritis
C. Renal stone
D. Trauma
E. Wilms tumour

19.4

In Johnathan's particular case (Question 19.3), what is the most likely organism to have been the cause of his previous urinary tract infections?

Select one answer only.

A. *Escherichia coli*
B. *Klebsiella* sp.
C. *Proteus* sp.
D. *Pseudomonas aeruginosa*
E. *Streptococcus faecalis*

19.5

Eesa, a 1-month-old Pakistani infant, is taken to his general practitioner by his mother. He is vomiting and not taking his feeds as well as normal. He is irritable and has a temperature of 39°C. His heart rate is 170 beats/min and his respiratory rate 45 breaths/min. The remainder of his examination is unremarkable. A clean catch urine sample is obtained and is positive for nitrites, leucocytes and protein on dipstick.

Which is the most appropriate next course of action?

Select one answer only.

A. Intravenous antibiotics
B. Intravenous fluids
C. Oral antibiotics
D. Oral paracetamol
E. Oral rehydration solution

19.6

Freddie is a 3-year-old boy. He is referred to the hospital as his mother has noticed that his face is swollen (Fig. 19.1). His mother was concerned that he had an allergic reaction to some peanuts he ate at a party. Examination reveals abdominal distension, bilateral scrotal swelling and pitting oedema of his lower limbs. Urine dipstick had 4+ protein, 2+ blood and nitrite and leucocyte negative. His blood pressure is normal for his age. You perform renal function tests, which reveal normal levels of sodium, potassium, urea, and creatinine. His complement levels (C3 and C4) are normal.

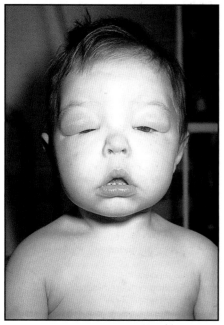

Figure 19.1

What is the most likely diagnosis?

Select one answer only.

A. Acute allergic reaction to peanuts
B. Acute glomerulonephritis
C. Haemolytic-uraemic syndrome
D. Nephrotic syndrome
E. Urinary tract infection

☞ **Hint: This child is losing lots of protein in his urine.**

19.7

What is the initial treatment of Freddie's condition?

Select one answer only.

A. Diuretics
B. Fluid restriction
C. Intravenous human albumin solution 20%
D. Intravenous hydrocortisone
E. Oral prednisolone

19.8

Finlay, a 5-year-old boy, recently had a birthday party at his local farm. Since then he has had 3 days of diarrhoea. The loose stool had some blood in it. His mother is concerned as he is still not himself. He appears to be very pale and has not passed urine for 12 hours. He has no other medical problems and is not normally on any medication. On examination you note that he has pale conjunctivae. His blood pressure is 120/70 mmHg. You decide to take some blood tests and get the following results:

- haemoglobin: 76 g/L; white blood cells: 14.2×10^9/L; platelet count: 50×10^9/L
- creatinine: 200 µmol/L (normal: 20–80 µmol/L)
- prothrombin time: 13 seconds (control: 12–15 s)
- activated partial thromboplastin time: 34 seconds (control: 25–35 s)

What is the most likely diagnosis?

Select one answer only.

A. Acute lymphatic leukaemia
B. Haemolytic-uraemic syndrome
C. Henoch–Schönlein purpura
D. Immune thrombocytopenic purpura
E. Post-streptococcal glomerulonephritis

19.9

Jane is a 5-year-old girl who presents to her general practice with bed-wetting. She has been wetting for 4 months and wets on average three nights per week. Her mother is upset as she had been dry during the day and night for almost a year. She recently started school and has had two episodes of wetting at school. She has no other medical problems and is not on any medication. She has always liked to drink water from a bottle she carries.

Which of the following would you do first?

Select one answer only.

A. Blood glucose
B. Ultrasound of the abdomen
C. Urinary dipstick
D. Urinary microscopy and culture
E. Water deprivation test

19.10

Hamza, a 14-year-old Indian boy, has chronic kidney disease secondary to renal dysplasia. His mother wants him to take more responsibility for his medication and would like you to talk to him about the different medicines he takes.

Which of the following dietary changes or medications is Hamza likely to be taking to prevent renal osteodystrophy?

Select one answer only.

A. Bicarbonate supplements
B. Calcium restriction
C. Phosphate supplements
D. Sodium supplements
E. Vitamin D supplements

Questions: Extended Matching

19.11

Below is a list of possible diagnoses (A–H) for which urinalysis may be undertaken. For each of the following patients who have urine microscopy and culture sent from the Emergency Department, select the most likely diagnosis. Each option may be used once, more than once, or not at all.

A. Balanitis
B. Glomerulonephritis
C. Nephrotic syndrome
D. Normal result
E. Perineal contamination
F. Renal stone (calculi)
G. Urinary tract infection
H. Vulvovaginitis

19.11.1

Ji is a 12-month-old Japanese girl who presents to the Emergency Department. She has a 2-day history of fever and vomiting. Her mother is concerned that she is dehydrated. On examination she is well hydrated and has marked coryza. She has an inflamed pharynx. A urine sample from a bag is sent to the laboratory. You obtain the following result from the microscopy and culture: white blood cells 100/mm^3; red blood cells negative; organisms, none seen; red cell casts, none seen; culture, not available.

19.11.2

Harriet, a 12-year-old girl, presents to the Emergency Department. She has abdominal pain and pain on micturition. A mid-stream urine sample is obtained and is positive for leucocytes but negative for nitrites. She was started on oral antibiotics and discharged; 48 hours later you receive the following result from the microscopy and culture: white blood cells >200/mm^3; red blood cells, many seen; organisms, none seen; red cell casts, none seen; culture, >10^5 coliforms.

19.11.3

Gary is a 6-month-old boy. He has been febrile for 1 day, is feeding poorly and has difficulty breathing. On examination he has a respiratory rate of 60 breaths/min, marked chest recession and on auscultation has widespread wheeze and fine crepitations. He needs admission for oxygen therapy.

A urine sample was sent from the Emergency Department and you receive the following results: white blood cells <50/mm^3; red blood cells, none seen; organisms, none seen; red cell casts, none seen; culture, mixed coliforms.

19.11.4

George is a 7-year-old boy who presents to his family doctor with cloudy urine. He has no other symptoms and his examination is normal. You obtain the following result from the microscopy and culture: white blood cells 50–100/mm^3; red blood cells, many seen; organisms, none seen; red cell casts seen; culture, negative at 48 hours.

19.11.5

Gregor is a 6-week-old baby who has recently moved to the UK from Estonia. He presents with fever and irritability. On examination he is clinically shocked. Because of the urgency to obtain a sample you take a catheter urine sample and start him immediately on intravenous antibiotics after a bolus of saline. You obtain the following result from the microscopy and culture: white blood cells >200/mm^3; red blood cells, none seen; organisms seen on microscopy; red cell casts not seen; culture >10^5 coliforms.

19.12

Below is a list (A–J) of renal investigations. For each of the following cases which investigation would you perform next? Each option may be used once, more than once, or not at all.

A. Antistreptolysin O titre
B. CT scan of the abdomen
C. DMSA scan
D. MAG3 renogram
E. Micturating cystourethrogram (MCUG)
F. Plain abdominal X-ray
G. Plasma creatinine and electrolytes
H. Ultrasound of the kidneys and urinary tract
I. Urinary electrolytes
J. Urine microscopy and culture

19.12.1

Max is a 12-year-old boy with cerebral palsy and epilepsy. He presents to the Emergency Department with severe right-sided colicky abdominal pain. He has had one episode of this previously, which ended as quickly as it started. Today the pain is so severe that he has needed morphine in the department. On examination you find a generally tender abdomen. He has a temperature of 37° C, heart rate of 160 beats/min, and his blood pressure is 120/80 mmHg. Urine dipstick has been performed and reveals haematuria.

19.12.2

Rosa, a 2-year-old girl, presents to her general practitioner. She has a 24-hour history of vomiting and fever. She has a temperature of 38° C. She has generalized tenderness of the abdomen. A dipstick reveals leucocytes and nitrites. Her blood pressure is 90/50 mmHg.

19.12.3

Usmaan is an 18-hour-old newborn baby boy who you are seeing for his routine discharge baby check. You read in his notes that he was found to have bilateral hydronephrosis and a distended bladder on his antenatal ultrasound scan. He mother is breastfeeding and does not feel she has started producing milk yet as

Usmaan has not passed urine. He has a normal blood pressure for a neonate.

19.12.4

John is a 9-year-old boy. He has a history of numerous urinary tract infections. He has had an ultrasound scan, which reveals that his kidneys are dysplastic. You are seeing him in the routine paediatric follow-up clinic. His mother does not feel he is growing as well as his siblings. His blood pressure is 130/90 mmHg.

Answers: Single Best Answer

19.1
A. Bag sample
A bag sample involves placing an adhesive plastic bag to the perineum after washing. This may also result in contamination from skin flora.

B. Catheter sample
A catheter sample can be obtained if there is urgency in obtaining a sample and no urine has recently been passed. However, it is invasive and can introduce infection.

C. Clean catch ⊘
Correct. This involves waiting with a sterile bowl to catch the urine. It is the least invasive and has less risk of contamination. The child is well enough to wait before starting treatment and you want to be sure that you are actually treating a urinary tract infection. The smell of urine is an unreliable sign of genuine infection.

D. Pad/cotton wool balls in nappy
A pad or cotton wool balls can be used in a nappy but risks contamination, resulting in a false-positive result.

E. Suprapubic aspirate
A suprapubic aspirate is sometimes used in severely ill infants requiring urgent diagnosis and treatment but it is invasive. It is increasingly replaced by urethral catheter sampling.

19.2
A. Appendicitis
The absence of abdominal tenderness makes appendicitis less likely.

B. Cystitis ⊘
Correct. She most likely has cystitis as she has urine frequency and abdominal pain.

C. Diabetic ketoacidosis
This must be considered. The urine must also be checked for glucose but it is a much less common diagnosis than lower urinary tract infection.

D. Glomerulonephritis
There would be dark brown urine or frank haematuria.

E. Pyelonephritis
As she does not have features of upper urinary tract infection, namely fever, feeling systemically unwell, localised abdominal or flank pain or tenderness, pyelonephritis is unlikely.

19.3
A. Constipation
He does not have a history of infrequent defaecation and the pain is unlikely to be so acute or severe.

B. Glomerulonephritis
Usually little or no pain and many red cells and often protein and leucocytes on urine analysis.

C. Renal stone ⊘
Correct. He is afebrile and the pain is spasmodic and severe. His previous urinary tract infections will have put him at higher risk of stone formation.

D. Trauma
There is no history of trauma.

E. Wilms tumour
Wilms tumour can present with flank pain and haematuria but a mass is usually palpable.

19.4
A. *Escherichia coli*
This is the most common organism to cause urinary tract infection but would not result in stone formation.

B. *Klebsiella* sp.
The second most common cause of urinary tract infection but does not result in stone formation.

C. *Proteus* sp. ⊘
Correct. *Proteus* infection predisposes to the formation of phosphate stones by splitting urea to ammonia and thus alkalinizing the urine. It is more commonly diagnosed in boys than in girls, possibly because of its presence under the prepuce.

D. *Pseudomonas aeruginosa*
Common only in children with indwelling catheters, when colonization can become chronic.

E. *Streptococcus faecalis*
A cause but rarer than the others listed.

19.5
A. Intravenous antibiotics ⊘
Correct. All infants less than 3 months old who are febrile and systemically unwell should be referred immediately to a paediatric department as they need treatment with intravenous antibiotics. He probably is septicaemic from a urinary tract infection as his urine is positive for nitrites, leucocytes and protein on dipstick. However, dipsticks should not be relied upon to diagnose urinary tract infection in children aged under 3 months; at this age, urine microscopy and culture should be used.

B. Intravenous fluids
Whilst he may require intravenous fluids, this will not effectively treat his urinary tract infection. A bolus of 0.9% saline is required if in shock.

C. Oral antibiotics
Oral antibiotics are suitable first-line treatment for children with uncomplicated urinary tract infection without evidence of serious bacterial infection.

D. Oral paracetamol
Children in pain should be given paracetamol or another analgesic agent. However, this should not delay treatment with antibiotics in this case.

E. Oral rehydration solution
Oral rehydration solution is an essential treatment for children with gastroenteritis who are dehydrated. This will not treat his urinary tract infection.

19.6

A. Acute allergic reaction to peanuts
In acute allergic reaction to peanuts there may be periorbital oedema but there is no generalized oedema.

B. Acute glomerulonephritis
In acute glomerulonephritis there may be periorbital oedema but there is no generalized oedema. Complement level would be low.

C. Haemolytic-uraemic syndrome
Expect marked pallor and possibly bloody stools if this is the diagnosis.

D. Nephrotic syndrome ⊘
Correct. This is the characteristic presentation. He will have very low serum albumin which leads to widespread capillary leak and fluid accumulation. He will have gained a significant amount of weight (from fluid).

E. Urinary tract infection
Not all dipstick-positive urine tests are the result of infection. The absence of nitrites and leucocytes makes infection unlikely. It would not result in generalized oedema.

19.7

A. Diuretics
Diuretics are not indicated at presentation in this child. They may be used with caution if fluid accumulation is causing significant symptoms (e.g. painful scrotal oedema).

B. Fluid restriction
Fluid restriction is not indicated in this child. In some instances, children with nephrotic syndrome become hypovolemic. Abdominal pain is often a feature and should prompt a thorough review.

C. Intravenous human albumin solution 20%
Human albumin solution is not indicated in this child. It is sometimes given for hypovolaemia or in steroid-resistant disease.

D. Intravenous hydrocortisone
Intravenous corticosteroids are not indicated.

E. Oral prednisolone ⊘
Correct. In 85% to 90% of children with nephrotic syndrome, the proteinuria resolves with corticosteroid therapy (steroid-sensitive nephrotic syndrome).

19.8

A. Acute lymphatic leukaemia
Acute lymphatic leukaemia can present with anaemia and thrombocytopenia; however, the other features of the history make this less likely.

B. Haemolytic-uraemic syndrome ⊘
Correct. This is a characteristic presentation with the triad of acute renal failure, microangiopathic haemolytic anaemia and thrombocytopenia. Typical haemolytic-uraemic syndrome is secondary to gastrointestinal infection with verocytotoxin-producing *Escherichia coli* O157:H7 acquired through contact with farm animals or eating uncooked beef, or, less often, *Shigella*.

C. Henoch–Schönlein purpura
Henoch–Schönlein purpura usually presents with a rash.

D. Immune thrombocytopenic purpura
Immune thrombocytopenic purpura presents with a purpuric rash.

E. Post-streptococcal glomerulonephritis
Post-streptococcal glomerulonephritis would present with acute nephritis after a streptococcal infection such as tonsillitis but would not be accompanied by anaemia and thrombocytopaenia.

19.9

A. Blood glucose
This would identify hyperglycaemia but is unnecessarily invasive with this history if the urine has no glucose in it.

B. Ultrasound of the abdomen
A useful non-invasive test but not the first line investigation.

C. Urinary dipstick ⊘
Correct. She has secondary enuresis, which is the loss of previously achieved urinary continence. A urine dipstick would be useful immediately as it would be abnormal if she had a urinary tract infection or diabetes. The urine dipstick helps guide one to further investigations. The likely cause is emotional upset from starting school and advice can be given once medical conditions have been ruled out.

D. Urinary microscopy and culture
A helpful test, but it would be prudent to dipstick the urine first as this would identify abnormalities suggestive of a urinary tract infection as well as glycosuria from diabetes and is easier to perform.

E. Water deprivation test
Diabetes insipidus is a rare diagnosis. If the symptoms persist and the urinalysis is normal, this may need to be excluded.

19.10
A. Bicarbonate supplements
Bicarbonate supplementation is required to prevent acidosis. This does not have a big effect on bone health though.

B. Calcium restriction
On the contrary, a high calcium diet is indicated as children with renal failure typically have low levels. This also helps to bind dietary phosphate, which otherwise would be absorbed and result in elevated phosphate levels.

C. Phosphate supplements
Phosphate intake should be restricted in children with chronic kidney disease.

D. Sodium supplements
Sodium supplements are sometimes needed in children with renal disease due to the loss of sodium into their urine but these do not prevent renal osteodystrophy.

E. Vitamin D supplements ⊘
Correct. Reduced activation of vitamin D results in secondary hyperparathyroidism, which causes phosphate retention and hypocalcaemia. Activated vitamin D supplements help prevent renal osteodystrophy.

Answers: Extended Matching

19.11.1
E. Perineal contamination
The number of white blood cells is mildly raised. This is most likely a false-positive result, from contamination of the sample. This occurs more often if the sample is not a clean catch. White cells from the skin, including the vagina in girls or foreskin in boys, are 'washed' into the sample as the urine waits in the bag. This is why a clean-catch sample is better.

Answer 19.11.2
G. Urinary tract infection
This girl had a 'false negative' on her dipstick test. The clinical story is very important for diagnosing urinary tract infection in this age group. The culture 48 hours later confirms the presence of coliforms in the urine.

Answer 19.11.3
E. Perineal contamination
This case highlights that our tests should be clinically guided. He presented with bronchiolitis

yet a urine sample was sent. Though he has a positive culture, it is a mixed growth and there is no pyuria (white cells in urine). This is a likely contaminant.

Answer 19.11.4
B. Glomerulonephritis
George has glomerulonephritis. The presence of red cell casts in the urine is always pathological. It is strongly indicative of glomerular damage.

Answer 19.11.5
G. Urinary tract infection
Gregor was systemically unwell on arrival and needed resuscitation. Sometimes a urine sample cannot be gained before starting antibiotics but in this case a catheter was employed.

Answer 19.12.1
H. Renal ultrasound
He is likely to have renal stones. Some anti-epileptic medications can increase the risk. The first-line investigation would be an ultrasound scan as this would usually demonstrate the site of obstruction and the presence of most stones (even radiolucent ones). Max's blood pressure and heart rate are mildly elevated. These should be re-checked once his pain is ameliorated.

Answer 19.12.2
J. Urine microscopy and culture
Urinary tract infection is the most likely diagnosis. In children under the age of 3 years, urine microscopy and culture should be used to diagnose urinary tract infection rather than urine dipstick alone.

Answer 19.12.3
H. Ultrsound of kidneys and urinary tract
This child needs an urgent ultrasound. Bilateral hydronephrosis on antenatal scanning can indicate urinary obstruction in the lower renal tract. Usmaan may have posterior urethral valves, which may be preventing him from voiding urine. If the ultrasound confirms bilateral hydronephrosis and/or a distended bladder, a MCUG (micturating cystourethrogram) would need to be performed prior to surgery. This management should be planned antenatally.

Answer 19.12.4
G. Plasma creatinine and electrolytes
John may be in renal failure and it is important to measure his renal function. The serum creatinine will be the most useful to identify chronic kidney disease. It is also important to know what his current serum potassium level is.

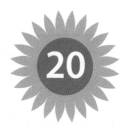
Genital disorders

20.1

Gary, a 2-month-old infant, is referred urgently to outpatients because of an intermittent swelling in both groins as shown in Fig. 20.1.

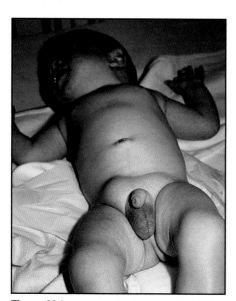

Figure 20.1

How would you best manage this child?

Select one answer only.

A. Needs immediate emergency surgical repair
B. Needs surgical repair promptly on next routine surgical list
C. Place on the waiting list for routine surgical repair
D. Reassess at 1 year of age to determine if surgery is still required
E. Reassure that this will resolve spontaneously

20.2 Testicular swelling

Jean-Paul, a 13-year-old boy, has developed an acutely painful red scrotum. On examination, his right testis is found to be swollen and lying higher in the scrotum than the left. It is tender on palpation.

What is the most important diagnosis to exclude?

Select one answer only.

A. Epididymitis
B. Hydrocele
C. Idiopathic scrotal oedema
D. Torsion of the appendage of the testes (hydatid of Morgagni)
E. Torsion of the testis

👆 **Hint: Which will lead to testicular loss if not diagnosed promptly?**

20.3

David, a 1-year-old infant, is brought to the Emergency Department by his mother because he has a swollen and red foreskin. It has become worse over the last few days and there is a discharge from the end of his penis. He has not suffered from anything like this before.

Which of the following represents the best treatment plan?

Select one answer only.

A. Broad-spectrum antibiotic and warm baths
B. Broad-spectrum antibiotics followed by circumcision
C. Circumcision on an elective list
D. Ice-cold baths
E. Immediate circumcision on the emergency list

20.4

Harry is a newborn infant. His parents have noticed that his genitalia look abnormal. Examination findings are shown in Fig. 20.2 below. Both testes are palpable.

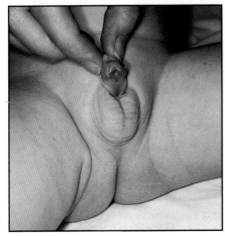

Figure 20.2

What management would you initiate?

Select one answer only.

A. Advise that surgery will be needed when older and will correct the problem
B. Advise that he is at an increased risk of other congenital abnormalities
C. Chromosomal analysis to check his gender
D. Reassure his parents that it is a variant of normal
E. Ultrasound of the bladder and kidneys

Answers: Single Best Answer

20.1

A. Needs immediate emergency surgical repair
This boy has bilateral inguinal hernias, which are present intermittently and therefore are reducible and do not pose an immediate threat to the contents of the hernia.

B. Needs surgical repair promptly on next routine surgical list ⊘
Correct. Repair should be done on the next routine operating list because of the risk of strangulation.

C. Place on the waiting list for routine surgical repair
The risk of strangulation is high in infants. Therefore surgery should be done promptly.

D. Reassess at 1 year of age to determine if surgery is still required
The hernia is due to a patent processus vaginalis, which will not close spontaneously. Surgery should be done promptly to avoid strangulation.

E. Reassure that this will resolve spontaneously
The hernia is due to a patent processus vaginalis, which will not close spontaneously. Therefore surgery is necessary.

20.2

A. Epididymitis
This diagnosis is not the most common or dangerous cause of an acute red scrotum in this age group.

B. Hydrocele
A hydrocele should not be red or present acutely.

C. Idiopathic scrotal oedema
This is not usually painful.

D. Torsion of the appendage of the testes (hydatid of Morgagni)
More common than torsion but not as dramatic clinical features. Usually before puberty.

E. Torsion of the testis ⊘
Correct. Surgical exploration is mandatory unless torsion can be excluded, because it must be relieved within 6–12 hours of the onset of symptoms for there to be a good chance of testicular viability.

20.3

A. Broad-spectrum antibiotic and warm baths ⊘
Correct. This boy is suffering from balanoposthitis. Treatment is with warm baths and a broad-spectrum antibiotic.

B. Broad-spectrum antibiotics followed by circumcision
The antibiotics will treat the condition, and circumcision will not be required.

C. Circumcision on an elective list
Circumcision is only indicated for recurrent balanoposthitis.

D. Ice-cold baths
There is active inflammation and infection, and this will not be treated by an ice-cold bath.

E. Immediate circumcision on the emergency list
This is balanoposthitis (inflammation of the glans and foreskin); recurrent attacks of balanoposthitis are uncommon, and only then is circumcision indicated.

20.4

A. Advise that surgery will be needed when older and will correct the problem ⊘
Correct. This is a glanular hypospadias. Surgery is performed to ensure that the boy can pass urine in a single stream in a straight line, has a straight penile shaft and straight erection and has a normal looking penis.

B. Advise that he is at an increased risk of other congenital abnormalities
Hypospadias affecting the glans is not associated with other congenital abnormalities.

C. Chromosomal analysis to check his gender
As both testes are descended and the phallus is of normal size, chromosomal analysis is not necessary.

D. Reassure his parents that it is a variant of normal
Hypospadias is a congenital structural abnormality of the urethra and meatus and is frequently associated with ventral curvature of the shaft of the penis and a hooded foreskin. It is not a variant of normal.

E. Ultrasound of the bladder and kidneys
Hypospadias is not associated with renal tract abnormalities unless very severe, so ultrasound of the kidneys and bladder is not indicated.

Liver disorders

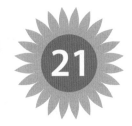

Questions: Single Best Answer

21.1
Manuel, a 3-day-old infant is born to healthy parents. He presents with oozing from the umbilical stump and sleepiness. On examination he is pale and grunting. He responds only to painful stimuli. He has marked hepatomegaly. Oxygen is delivered and senior help summoned as he is very unwell. The nurse practitioner inserts an intravenous line and asks what blood tests you would like first.

From the following list of blood tests pick the one you would undertake first.

Select one answer only.

A. Ammonia
B. Blood culture
C. Blood gas
D. Blood glucose
E. Coagulation studies

21.2.
Reece, a 4-week-old male infant living in the UK, is taken to his family doctor because he is jaundiced. He was born at term and is breastfed. His mother reports that he has always looked yellow and has started to develop bruises. His stools are now pale in colour. On examination he has hepatomegaly.

Which of the following investigations would you undertake first?

Select one answer only.

A. Faecal elastase
B. Serum conjugated and unconjugated bilirubin
C. Sweat test
D. Ultrasound scan of the liver
E. Urinalysis

21.3.
Javid is a 5-month-old Asian baby born at term in rural Pakistan. He presents with jaundice. His mother's blood group is AB rhesus positive. His stool and urine are a normal colour. He is breastfed, although he has not been feeding well. His mother is concerned that this could be due to his constipation. When you examine the infant (Fig. 21.1) you note that he has dry skin and an umbilical hernia.

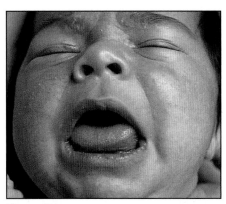

Figure 21.1

Which of the following is the most likely diagnosis?

Select one answer only.

A. Biliary atresia
B. Congenital infection
C. Galactosaemia
D. Rhesus haemolytic disease of the newborn
E. Hypothyroidism

21.4.
Luna, a 32-year-old Cantonese woman has just given birth to her third child. She arrived in the UK 3 months ago to live with her extended family following the death of her husband. Antenatal screening shows that she is hepatitis B surface antigen (HBsAg) positive and hepatitis B e antigen (HBeAg) negative. The newborn infant looks well and has fed. The postnatal team are keen to send the mother and baby home.

Which of the following is the best advice to give concerning immunization of the family?

Select one answer only.

A. Hepatitis B vaccination for the baby
B. Hepatitis B vaccination for the baby and all other children
C. Hepatitis B vaccination for the baby and mother
D. Hepatitis B vaccination for the baby with hepatitis B immunoglobulin
E. No treatment required

21.5.
Summer, a 12-year-old girl, is seen in the Emergency Department. Her parents report that her school performance has been deteriorating and recently she has become confused and unsteady on her feet.

Examination findings of her eyes are shown in Fig. 21.2.

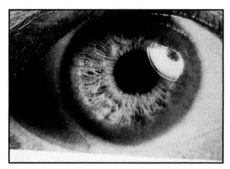

Figure 21.2 (Courtesy of Prof Deidre Kelly).

Select the most likely diagnosis.

Select one answer only.

A. Glaucoma
B. Hyperthyroidism
C. Illicit drug use
D. Intracranial tumour
E. Wilson disease

Questions: Extended Matching

21.6.
The following is a list of diagnoses (A–L). For each of the following patients with liver disease, select the most likely diagnosis from the list. Each option may be used once, more than once, or not at all.

A. α_1-antitrypsin deficiency
B. Autoimmune hepatitis
C. Bacterial infection
D. Biliary atresia
E. Cystic fibrosis
F. Hepatitis A
G. Hepatitis B
H. Hepatitis C
I. Inflammatory bowel disease
J. Galactosaemia
K. Primary sclerosing cholangitis
L. Wilson disease

21.6.1.
Jason, a 3-week-old boy, is still jaundiced. His mother is reassured that this is likely to be 'breast milk' jaundice as she is fully breastfeeding him. He presents 3 weeks later with poor feeding, vomiting and bruising on his forehead and limbs. He has pale stools. On examination the liver is palpable 4 cm below the costal margin.

21.6.2.
Raj, a previously well 14-year-old Asian boy, is noted to be jaundiced. He has recently returned to the UK from India where he was visiting relatives in a rural village. He had a 10-day diarrhoea and vomiting illness whilst in India.

21.6.3.
A 5-week-old southern Asian male infant born in the UK presents to the Paediatric Assessment Unit with vomiting. He has not gained weight since birth. On examination you find an infant who is jaundiced, lethargic and hypotonic. Cataracts are present.

21.6.4.
Lee is a 12-year-old Chinese boy who moved with his parents from China 2 years ago. He presents with episodes of vomiting which is blood-stained. On examination he is jaundiced, malnourished and has splenomegaly.

Answers: Single Best Answer

21.1

A. Ammonia
Manuel may have liver failure and high ammonia. However, knowing this will not help your initial management.

B. Blood culture
There may be infection here and blood cultures are indicated. However, failure to do so will not change initial management.

C. Blood gas
This is almost certain to demonstrate a marked acidosis. In practice it may give a blood glucose measurement too but a blood gas is not the priority.

D. Blood glucose ⊘
Correct. This must be done. Hypoglycaemia is an important consequence of serious illness including liver failure, e.g. from galactosaemia in view of his hepatomegaly and bleeding and sepsis. The priorities for management are:
- maintain blood glucose
- treat sepsis with broad-spectrum antibiotics
- prevent haemorrhage with intravenous vitamin K and fresh frozen plasma.

E. Coagulation studies
Important but likely to be deranged as there is bleeding.

21.2

A. Faecal elastase
A useful test to determine exocrine pancreatic insufficiency, but not the priority here.

B. Serum conjugated and unconjugated bilirubin ⊘
Correct. This will enable you to identify whether, as the history suggests, this child has a conjugated hyperbilirubinaemia. If this is the case then urgent further investigation is necessary as the child may have biliary atresia. Delay in diagnosis and definitive treatment adversely affects outcome.

C. Sweat test
Reece should have had a screening test for cystic fibrosis at birth. It may cause prolonged conjugated jaundice but is not a first-line investigation.

D. Ultrasound scan of the liver
This can help identify the likely underlying cause. A fasting abdominal ultrasound scan may demonstrate an absent or shrunken gallbladder in biliary atresia but one first needs to confirm conjugated jaundice.

E. Urinalysis
The urine is likely to be dark if the child has neonatal liver disease. However, laboratory testing is not usually necessary.

21.3

A. Biliary atresia
Biliary atresia is very unlikely here due to the normal stool colour. However, a blood test to assess the proportion of conjugated bilirubin should be performed. If this is raised, then biliary atresia would be considered.

B. Congenital infection
The TORCH congenital infections (*toxoplasmosis, syphilis, rubella, cytomegalovirus,* or *herpes*) are acquired by the mother during pregnancy and passed on to the developing fetus. Affected babies may be jaundiced, but they characteristically have other problems of the heart, skin, eye, and central nervous system.

C. Galactosaemia
Galactosaemia is a rare disorder of carbohydrate metabolism that presents with poor feeding, vomiting, jaundice and hepatomegaly when fed milk.

D. Rhesus haemolytic disease of the newborn
Not the cause as the mother is AB rhesus positive. Rhesus disease could be possible if the mother was rhesus negative. ABO incompatibility is usually only seen in mothers with an O blood group.

E. Hypothyroidism ⊘
Correct. Hypothyroidism is a cause of prolonged jaundice in infants. Clinical features include dry skin, constipation, coarse facial features including a large tongue as in the figure, umbilical hernia and a hoarse cry. In the UK it is usually identified on newborn biochemical screening (Guthrie test).

21.4

A. Hepatitis B vaccination for the baby
This is required but it is important to also vaccinate other family members (in this case the older siblings).

B. Hepatitis B vaccination for the baby and all other children ⊘
Correct. Prevention of hepatitis B virus infection is important. All pregnant women should have antenatal screening for HBsAg. Babies of all HBsAg-positive mothers should receive a course of hepatitis B vaccination (given routinely in many countries).

C. Hepatitis B vaccination for the baby and mother
The other children in the family should be vaccinated.

D. Hepatitis B vaccination for the baby with hepatitis B immunoglobulin
Hepatitis B immunoglobulin is also given if the mother is also HBeAg-positive. Antibody response to the vaccination course should be checked in high-risk infants at 12 months as 5% require further vaccination.

E. No treatment required
Incorrect. Approximately 30% to 50% of carrier children will develop chronic hepatitis B virus liver disease.

21.5

A. Glaucoma
Blurred vision and a sore eye or unilateral headache should make you consider glaucoma. It is a rare diagnosis in children but important not to miss.

B. Hyperthyroidism
This may cause reduced concentration at school and proptosis. However, the upper margin of the iris is not exposed here. Assessment for tachycardia/sweating will be required.

C. Illicit drug use
A cause of deterioration in school performance. Teenagers may also become secretive and withdrawn. Cannabis use may result in red eyes with dilated pupils. However, this is not what is shown.

D. Intracranial tumour
Eye signs are a common but rather late sign of brain tumours. The most obvious is a 'false-localizing sign' of VI nerve palsy. This results in double-vision and a failure to fully abduct the affected eye. Early morning headache and head tilt are both 'red-flag' signs.

E. Wilson disease ⊘
Correct. You are being shown Kayser-Fleischer rings from copper in the cornea. This is a very rare but treatable cause of liver failure/neurological deterioration. Neuropsychiatric features are more common in those presenting from the second decade onwards and include deterioration in school performance, mood and behaviour change and extrapyramidal signs such as incoordination, tremor and dysarthria. A very rare diagnosis – a typical hospital in the UK will see one case every 30 years (it has an incidence of 1 in 200 000).

Answers: Extended Matching

Answer 21.6.1
D. Biliary atresia
All infants with jaundice after 2 weeks of age should be investigated to exclude this. The parents should never be reassured that this is breast milk related until a conjugated bilirubin has been shown to be normal. The pale stool occurs due to failure of the liver to excrete bile, and indicates that the jaundice is conjugated, and therefore not due to breast milk jaundice.

Answer 21.6.2
F. Hepatitis A
Hepatitis A virus. Vaccination is recommended for those travelling to endemic areas but it incurs a charge and many families do not undertake it.

Answer 21.6.3
J. Galactosaemia
In this very rare disorder infants develop poor feeding, vomiting, jaundice and hepatomegaly when fed milk. Liver failure, cataracts and developmental delay are inevitable if untreated. A rapidly fatal course with shock and disseminated intravascular coagulation, often due to Gram-negative sepsis, may occur. For this reason, galactosaemia is being screened for in some countries (but not the UK).
A bacterial infection (such as a urinary tract infection) would need to be excluded.

Answer 21.6.4
G. Hepatitis B
Hepatitis B virus has a high prevalence and carrier rate in the Far East and sub-Saharan Africa. This child probably acquired the infection vertically from his mother or horizontally from another family member. His vomiting blood most likely represents oesophageal varices from portal hypertension. The main clue to hepatitis B is his country of origin.

Malignant disease

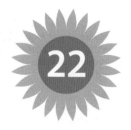

22.1
Concerning the epidemiology of childhood cancer, which of the following types is most common in the UK?

Select one answer only.

A. Bone tumour
B. Brain tumour
C. Leukaemia
D. Neuroblastoma
E. Wilms tumour (nephroblastoma)

22.2
Polly is a 2-year-old girl who is receiving chemotherapy for her acute lymphoblastic leukaemia. She is known to be neutropenic and has developed a fever of over 38.5°C.

What is the most appropriate course of action?

Select one answer only.

A. Be admitted to hospital for observation
B. Be started immediately on oral antibiotics
C. Have her blood count and inflammatory markers (e.g. C-reactive protein) measured
D. Have blood cultures taken and be started on intravenous antibiotics
E. See her general practitioner for further assessment and decision regarding antibiotics

22.3
Mohammed is a 3-year-old boy who is reviewed in the Paediatric Assessment Unit. He has a history of weight loss and lethargy. His mother is also concerned as he keeps crying and complains of pain in his tummy. On examination of his abdomen he has an extensive mass. The doctor is worried he may have a childhood malignancy.

Which of the following investigations would be the most useful in making the diagnosis?

Select one answer only.

A. Plasma ammonia
B. Plasma LDG (lactate dehydrogenase)
C. Serum α-fetoprotein
D. Serum beta-HCG (human chorionic gonadotrophin)
E. Urinary catecholamines

22.4
Josh is a 2-year-old boy who presents to the Emergency Department with weight loss and lethargy. On examination he has splenomegaly. You are worried that he has leukaemia. You perform an urgent full blood count.

What are the most likely haematology results if he has leukaemia?

Select one answer only.

A. Low haemoglobin and low platelets
B. High haemoglobin and low platelets
C. Normal haemoglobin and normal platelets
D. High haemoglobin and raised platelets
E. Low haemoglobin and raised platelets

22.5
Amy is a 2-year-old girl who presents to the outpatient department with a history of developmental regression. She was able to walk but has 'gone off her legs' in the last few weeks. Her parents are very worried about her. On further questioning she had been well with no preceding coryzal illness. On examination, she is very unsteady on her feet and her power is reduced in her lower limbs. She has no obvious visual problems and seems able to follow the picture book her mother has brought to clinic. A CT scan is obtained and is shown below in Fig. 22.1.

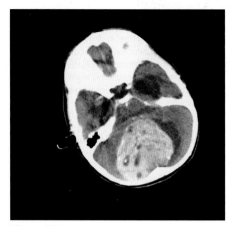

Figure 22.1

What is the most likely underlying cause?

Select one answer only.

A. Cerebral abscess
B. Cortical astrocytoma
C. Craniopharyngioma
D. Medulloblastoma
E. Viral encephalitis

22.6
Mark, a 3-year-old boy, is currently receiving chemotherapy. His sister has developed the rash shown in Fig. 22.3 below. Mark is well and does not have a fever.

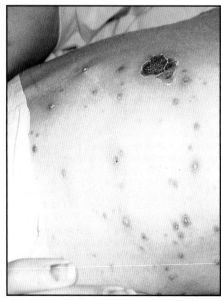

Figure 22.3

Mark's parents are worried and phone the oncology ward for advice.

What information should they be given?

Select one answer only.

A. Advise them to see their general practitioner to check that he is all right
B. Mark needs urgent treatment to prevent him from becoming unwell
C. Monitor Mark and if he becomes unwell with a fever, bring him to the ward
D. Monitor Mark and if he has any signs of the rash, bring him to the ward
E. Reassurance – this is a common illness that most children get

22.7
Essa is a 2-year-old boy whose parents have noticed his two eyes look different. He has no other medical history and is not currently on any medication. On examination, the movement of the eyes is normal and the pupils are equal and reactive to light. On checking his pupillary reflex you observe his left pupil looks red but the right looks white. His systemic examination is normal.

What is the likely cause of this?

Select one answer only.

A. Congenital cataract
B. Glaucoma
C. Retinoblastoma
D. Allergic conjunctivitis
E. VI nerve palsy

22.8
Brittney, aged 5 years, goes to her optician. She has needed glasses for 4 months but her mother thinks her prescription needs changing as she has been getting progressively worsening headaches. When the optician examines her eyes she finds the examination shown in Fig. 22.4. Both her eyes have a red reflex.

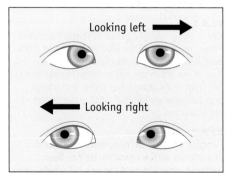

Figure 22.4

What is the most likely diagnosis?

Select one answer only.

A. Craniopharyngioma
B. Concomitant squint
C. Optic glioma
D. Posterior fossa tumour
E. Retinoblastoma

Questions: Extended Matching

22.9
Below is a list (A–K) of possible diagnoses. For each of the clinical scenarios, select the most likely diagnosis. Each option may be used once, more than once, or not at all.

A. Acute lymphoblastic leukaemia
B. Bone tumour
C. Brain tumour
D. Burkitt lymphoma
E. Henoch–Schönlein purpura
F. Hodgkin disease
G. Immune thrombocytopenia purpura
H. Langerhans cell histiocytosis
I. Neuroblastoma
J. Retinoblastoma
K. Wilms tumour (nephroblastoma)

22.9.1
Natalia, a 4-year-old girl, presents to her general practitioner. This is her second bad episode of tonsillitis in the same month. She is tired and looks pale and has a number of bruises on her lower legs. On examination she has pallor, scattered purpuric skin lesions and hepatosplenomegaly.

22.9.2
Angel, a 2-year-old boy, presents to his general practitioner with an abdominal mass noticed by his mother on dressing him. He has no other medical problems and is not on any medication. His stool pattern is regular. He is otherwise relatively well in himself. You examine his abdomen and feel a mass in his left abdomen, which does not cross the midline. There is no hepatosplenomegaly.

22.9.3
Kay, a 3-year-old girl, presents to the Paediatric Assessment Unit as her mother is worried she is pale, tired and 'not quite right'. She has also lost 2 kg of weight in the last month. On examination the child looks unwell, has pallor and a large firm, irregular abdominal mass in the centre of her abdomen.

22.9.4
Douglas, a 7-year-old boy, visits his general practitioner with his mother. He has been getting headaches over the last 3–5 weeks which

have increased in intensity. These have woken him from sleep. His mother reports that he has recently begun vomiting in the morning. His teachers have also commented his school work is getting worse. His mother thinks this may be because his sight has deteriorated as he keeps complaining of double vision.

22.10
Below is a list (A–K) of investigations. For each of the following patients with malignant disease select the investigation most likely to confirm the diagnosis. Each option may be used once, more than once, or not at all.

A. Bone marrow aspirate
B. Blood film
C. Chest X-ray
D. Clotting screen
E. CT scan
F. Excision biopsy
G. Full blood count
H. Magnetic resonance imaging (MRI) scan
I. Positron emission tomography (PET) scan
J. Ultrasound of abdomen
K. Urine catecholamines

22.10.1
Connor, a 4-year-old boy, presents to the Paediatric Assessment Unit with his parents. They are worried as he seems to be very tired and complains of his legs hurting. He also seems to have a fine rash that has developed on his arms. On examination he is pale, has a petechial rash on his arms and legs and has hepatosplenomegaly. A full blood count shows low haemoglobin and platelet count.

22.10.2
Niamh, a 4-year-old girl, is taken to her general practitioner as her mother has noticed she has red urine. On further questioning she has been more tired than normal and has been complaining of abdominal pain. On examination she is pale with a left-sided abdominal mass. Her urine is red and a dipstick confirms that this is blood.

22.10.3
Oscar, a 3-year-old boy, attends the Emergency Department as his mother is worried he has lost weight and looks pale. On examination he has a large irregular mass extending across his abdomen. His blood pressure is high.

22.10.4
Francis, a 2-year-old boy, is taken to his general practitioner by his father who is worried as he has become 'cross-eyed'. Otherwise he is very well in himself and has no history of vomiting. On examination he appears to be well but has an absent red reflex in his left eye.

22.10.5

Carla is a 4-year-old girl who is seen in the Paediatric Assessment Unit complaining of headaches. Her mother has noticed that her eye movements are not normal. The whole family has recently had a sickness bug but Carla seems to have continued vomiting.

22.10.6

Solomon is a 12-year-old boy. He has recently lost weight and his 'glands are up'. His mother reports that the 'glands' in his neck have been enlarged for several months now. He has no other medical problems. He has not been having any episodes of fever or night sweats. On examination he has several large, irregular, hard lymph nodes in his neck. They are all greater than 2 cm in size. You order a full blood count and blood film, which show normal results.

Answers: Single Best Answer

22.1
A. Bone tumour
Bone tumours represent about 4% of the total. They are uncommon before puberty. In adolescents they are an important cancer type and outcomes are not as good as those for leukaemia.

B. Brain tumour
Brain and spinal tumours make up about one-quarter of all childhood malignancies (24%). They often present late and treatment is difficult.

C. Leukaemia ⊘
Correct. Leukaemia is the most common malignancy in childhood (about a third of all cases; see Fig. 22.1 in Illustrated Textbook of Paediatrics). Acute lymphoblastic leukaemia is most likely. It accounts for 80% of leukaemia in children.

D. Neuroblastoma
This is a relatively rare tumour after the first 5 years of life but is a fairly common type in children under the age of 5 years. It makes up about 7% of the total.

E. Wilms tumour (nephroblastoma)
This is a rare tumour but affects a relatively narrow age range, being more common in children under 5 years of age and rarely seen after 10 years of age. Most children look remarkably well and may present with either an abdominal mass or haematuria.

22.2
A. Be admitted to hospital for observation
Children with febrile neutropenia become very unwell very quickly. This is a case where it is important to treat early and before overwhelming sepsis takes hold.

B. Be started immediately on oral antibiotics
Oral antibiotics are insufficient protection against the wide range of potential pathogens. Broad-spectrum intravenous antibiotics are required.

C. Have her blood count and inflammatory markers (e.g. C-reactive protein) measured
This would be done, but is not likely to change treatment. The main purpose of blood tests in this instance is to determine whether the child is neutropenic.

D. Have blood cultures taken and be started on intravenous antibiotics ⊘
Correct. Children with fever and neutropenia are at high risk of serious infection and must be admitted promptly to hospital for cultures and treatment with broad-spectrum antibiotics. The absence of neutrophils may lead to less obvious clinical signs than otherwise expected.

Merely observing or just giving oral antibiotics would not be aggressive enough for what could be a life-threatening infection.

E. See her general practitioner for further assessment and decision regarding antibiotics
This would add delay to the process of initiating appropriate treatment.

22.3
A. Plasma ammonia
Useful for the diagnosis of urea cycle disorders but not elevated in neuroblastoma.

B. Plasma LDG (lactate dehydrogenase)
Elevated (often significantly) in lymphoma and other solid tumours. Rather non-specific though, and will be increased in any process where there is increased cell breakdown, e.g. haemolysis.

C. Serum α-fetoprotein
Along with β-human chorionic gonadotropin, this is elevated in germ-cell tumours. However, these are rare.

D. Serum β-HCG (human chorionic gonadotrophin)
Along with α-fetoprotein, β-HCG is elevated in germ-cell tumours.

E. Urinary catecholamines ⊘
Correct. An extensive abdominal mass in an unwell child of his age suggests neuroblastoma. Urinary catecholamine levels would be elevated.

22.4
A. Low haemoglobin and low platelets ⊘
Correct. A low haemoglobin and low platelet count are often present at diagnosis due to bone marrow failure. Circulating leukaemic blast cells may be present. There is often either a very high or a low white cell count.

B. High haemoglobin and low platelets
Thrombocytopenia is common as is a high white cell count but there is normally an associated anaemia.

C. Normal haemoglobin and normal platelets
This can occur in the early stages. However, by the time there is splenomegaly this is unlikely.

D. High haemoglobin and raised platelets
This does not occur.

E. Low haemoglobin and raised platelets
A thrombocytosis is sometimes seen in chronic blood loss states or following viral infection. However, it is an unusual presenting feature of leukaemia.

22.5
A. Cerebral abscess
The clinical history usually gives a fever and there would be a 'ring enhancing lesion' on CT (or MRI) scan.

B. Cortical astrocytoma
Cortical astrocytoma is not likely as there is no evidence of raised intracranial pressure or focal neurological signs or seizures typical of cortical tumours and the mass is in the posterior fossa.

C. Craniopharyngioma
Craniopharyngioma is unlikely as there is no evidence of pituitary deficiency or visual field loss and the mass is in the posterior fossa.

D. Medulloblastoma ⊘
Correct. Medulloblastoma (~20% of brain tumours) arises in the midline of the posterior fossa (Fig. 22.2). These children present with truncal ataxia and incoordination.

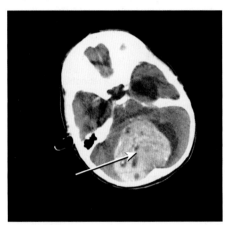

Figure 22.2

E. Viral encephalitis
Unlikely as there is no fever and she has ataxia and reduced power only of the lower limbs. The imaging also shows a mass.

22.6
A. Advise them to see their general practitioner to check that he is all right
This merely adds delay to the process. Nearly all children undergoing chemotherapy have open access to the ward.

B. Mark needs urgent treatment to prevent him from becoming unwell ⊘
Correct. His sister has varicella zoster (chicken pox) infection, and this can be life-threatening in immunocompromised patients. He needs treatment with varicella zoster immunoglobulin unless he is immune. The incubation period for varicella is 14–21 days, so one cannot be reassured by the fact that he is currently well.

C. Monitor Mark and if he becomes unwell with a fever, bring him to the ward
This is not appropriate as his sibling has chickenpox and the aim is to prevent him from becoming seriously ill from catching it.

D. Monitor Mark and if he has any signs of the rash, bring him to the ward
This is not appropriate as his sibling has chickenpox and the aim is to prevent him from becoming seriously ill from catching it.

E. Reassurance – this is a common illness that most children get
It is very dangerous in children who are receiving chemotherapy.

22.7
A. Cataract
Congenital cataract can cause leukocoria but would have been detected at an earlier age.

B. Glaucoma
Whilst this is a rare disease in childhood, it would be most likely to lead to a swollen red eye. There is often excess tear production and light sensitivity in children. It is more common in children with neurofibromatosis or Sturge–Weber syndrome.

C. Retinoblastoma ⊘
Correct. White papillary reflex (also known as leukocoria, see Fig. 22.17 in Illustrated Textbook of Paediatrics) requires urgent ophthalmological assessment as it can be caused by:
- retinoblastoma
- corneal opacity
- congenital cataract (usually presents shortly after birth)
- vitreous opacity
- retinal disease, e.g. retinal detachment.

There is no history of trauma or a foreign body making this unlikely.

D. Allergic conjunctivitis
Would cause bilateral conjunctivitis rather than a unilateral white reflex.

E. VI nerve palsy
A VI nerve palsy would not cause a white papillary reflex.

22.8
A. Craniopharyngioma
Craniopharyngioma can cause loss of visual fields, classically bitemporal hemianopia, rather than a VI nerve palsy.

B. Concomitant squint
This is a paralytic squint and not a concomitant (non-paralytic) squint.

C. Optic glioma
An optic glioma would affect vision but not the eye movements.

D. Posterior fossa tumour ⊘
Correct. Brittney has bilateral VI nerve palsy – she is unable to look to her left or right because of lateral abducens (VI) nerve palsy. She is likely to have a posterior fossa tumour. It is a false localizing sign from raised intracranial pressure.

E. Retinoblastoma
Retinoblastomas cause a white reflex but do not affect the eye movements.

Answers: Extended Matching

Answer 22.9.1
A. Acute lymphoblastic leukaemia
Clinical symptoms and signs result from disseminated disease and systemic ill health from infiltration of the bone marrow or other organs with leukaemic blast cells. In most children, leukaemia presents insidiously over several weeks but in some it presents and progresses very rapidly.

Answer 22.9.2
K. Wilms tumour (nephroblastoma)
Most children present in this way and before 5 years of age.

Answer 22.9.3
I. Neuroblastoma
Most common before 5 years of age and most children present with an abdominal mass, which is large and complex, crossing the midline. Over the age of 2 years, clinical symptoms are mostly from metastatic disease, particularly bone pain, bone marrow suppression causing weight loss and malaise.

Answer 22.9.4
C. Brain tumour
The HeadSmart campaign (www.headsmart .org.uk) highlights presentation of brain tumours in children of his age:
  • persistent/recurrent headaches
  • persistent/recurrent vomiting
  • abnormal balance/walking/coordination
  • abnormal eye movements, blurred or double vision
  • behaviour change
  • seizures
  • abnormal head position, e.g. head tilt, wry neck, stiff neck.

Answer 22.10.1
A. Bone marrow aspirate
This child has most likely got acute lymphoblastic leukaemia. A full blood count and blood film would be very useful but to confirm and classify the diagnosis a bone marrow examination is essential.

Answer 22.10.2
J. Ultrasound of abdomen
This child is likely to have a Wilms tumour (nephroblastoma). An ultrasound is the easiest test to perform and so would be performed prior to either a CT or MRI scan.

Answer 22.10.3
K. Urine catecholamines
This child is likely to have a neuroblastoma. Urinary catecholamine levels would be raised. A confirmatory biopsy is usually obtained and evidence of metastatic disease is detected with bone marrow sampling and MIBG (metaiodobenzylguanidine) scan with or without a bone scan.

Answer 22.10.4
H. MRI scan
This child is likely to have a retinoblastoma and this is best confirmed using a MRI scan of the head and an eye examination under anaesthesia.

Answer 22.10.5
H. MRI scan
This child is likely to have a brain tumour. Brain tumours are best characterized on MRI scan. Often a CT scan is performed first if MRI is not readily available, but is not as good at identifying tumour type. Magnetic resonance spectroscopy can be used to examine the biological activity of a tumour. Lumbar puncture must not be performed without neurosurgical advice if there is any suspicion of raised intracranial pressure.

Answer 22.10.6
F. Excision biopsy
It is common for children to have cervical lymphadenopathy, but here the warning signs are weight loss and large and irregular lymph nodes. The concern is that this boy has a lymphoma. A normal full blood count and blood film cannot rule out the diagnosis and a lymph node biopsy would have to be performed.

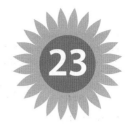

Haematological disorders

Questions: Single Best Answer

23.1

Tia is a 4-year-old Caucasian girl. She is referred to the paediatric ward by her general practitioner as her mother noted that she had a yellow tinge to her eyes since developing an upper respiratory tract infection. She is well in herself and has no history of weight loss. There is no family history of any blood disorders. On examination she was pale and her spleen was enlarged 3 cm below the costal margin.

You perform a full blood count, which reveals:
- Hb (haemoglobin): 60 g/L
- WBC (white blood cell count): 8×10^9/L
- platelet count: 255×10^9/L
- blood film: small red cells
- MCV (mean cell volume): 60 fL (normal: 75–87 fL)

What is the most likely diagnosis?

Select one answer only.

A. Acute lymphoblastic leukaemia
B. Glucose-6-phosphate dehydrogenase (G6PD) deficiency
C. Hereditary spherocytosis
D. Sickle cell disease
E. Thalassaemia

23.2

Ahmed, whose parents come from Egypt, is a 10-year-old boy who presents to his general practitioner. This evening he is more lethargic than usual and his urine has become dark in colour. There is no history of excessive exercise or beetroot consumption; in fact, they had a festive meal of chicken, fish, broad beans and rice for lunch. His examination is normal and he is afebrile. He has no medical history of note. He has not had a recent upper respiratory tract infection.

What is the most likely underlying cause of his new symptoms?

Select one answer only.

A. Acute lymphatic leukaemia
B. β-Thalassaemia trait
C. G6PD (Glucose-6-phosphate dehydrogenase) deficiency
D. Pyelonephritis
E. Sickle cell disease

23.3

Tom is a 5-year-old boy who presents to hospital with a recent history of bruising easily. Two weeks ago he had an upper respiratory tract infection which resolved spontaneously. On examination today he is afebrile but has many, widespread bruises with some scattered petechiae.

Investigations reveal:
- Hb (haemoglobin): 116 g/L
- WBC (white blood cell count): 10.2×10^9/L
- platelet count: 32×10^9/L
- prothrombin time: 15 seconds (control: 12–15 s)
- activated partial thromboplastin time: 30 seconds (control: 25–35 s)
- fibrinogen: 2.5 g/L (normal: 2–4 g/L)

What is the most likely diagnosis?

Select one answer only.

A. Acute lymphoblastic leukaemia
B. Haemophilia A
C. Immune thrombocytopenic purpura
D. Non-accidental injury
E. Vitamin D deficiency

23.4

Amir is a 2-year-old Bangladeshi boy who has eczema. His general practitioner is undertaking a routine review of his care and notices that Amir is pale. The remainder of his examination is normal. His mother reports that he has been eating bits of carpet from his room recently.

Investigations reveal:

- Hb (haemoglobin): 66 g/L
- WBC (white blood cell count): 10.2×10^9/L
- platelet count: 350×10^9/L
- MCV (mean cell volume): 60 fL (normal: 75–87 fL)

What is the most appropriate treatment?

Select one answer only.

A. Dietary advice
B. Folic acid
C. Iron supplements
D. Multivitamin tablets
E. Vitamin B_{12} injections

23.5

Joseph, a 2-year-old black Caribbean boy from London, is admitted to hospital for an elective repair of an inguinal hernia. He has no other medical problems. His pre-operative assessment reveals the following results and his blood film is shown below (Fig. 23.1):

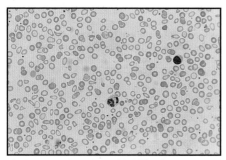

Figure 23.1 (Courtesy of Prof Paula Bolton-Maggs).

- Hb (haemoglobin): 86 g/L
- MCV (mean cell volume): 68 fL (normal: 75–87 fL)
- MCHC (mean corpuscular haemoglobin concentration): 22 g/dl (normal: 32–35 g/dl)
- WBC (white blood cell count): 11.2×10^9/L
- platelets: 262×10^9/L
- HB electrophoresis: haemoglobin A (HbA) 98%; haemoglobin A_2 (HbA_2) 2%

What is the most likely diagnosis?

Select one answer only.

A. β-Thalassaemia trait
B. Glucose-6-phosphate dehydrogenase deficiency
C. Iron-deficiency anaemia
D. Normal variation for age and ethnicity
E. Sickle cell trait

23.6

Peter, aged 9 months, presents to the Emergency Department. His family moved to the UK when Peter was 6 weeks old. He has a 6 hour history of pain in his fingers. He has had an upper respiratory tract infection for the past 24 hours. He has no other medical history and is not on any medication.

The appearance of his left hand is shown in Fig. 23.2. What is the most likely diagnosis?

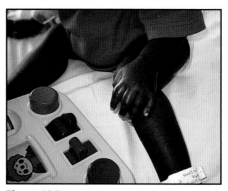

Figure 23.2

Select one answer only.

A. Acute lymphoblastic leukaemia
B. β-Thalassaemia major
C. Glucose-6-phosphate dehydrogenase deficiency
D. Haemophilia A
E. Sickle cell disease

Questions: Extended Matching

23.7

Below is a list of possible diagnoses (A–R). For each of the following patients with haematological problems select the most likely diagnosis. Each option may be used once, more than once, or not at all.

A. Acute lymphoblastic leukaemia
B. Acute myeloid leukaemia
C. α-Thalassaemia major
D. α-Thalassaemia trait
E. β-Thalassaemia major
F. β-Thalassaemia trait
G. Glucose-6-phosphate dehydrogenase deficiency
H. Haemophilia A
I. Immune thrombocytopenic purpura
J. Infectious mononucleosis
K. Iron deficiency anaemia
L. Liver disease
M. Meningococcal disease

N. Normal variant
O. Sickle cell disease
P. Vitamin D deficiency
Q. Vitamin K deficiency
R. von Willebrand disease

23.7.1
Shlomo is a 9-day-old Jewish boy who was born in the UK. He had a religious circumcision yesterday, but the wound will not stop bleeding. On examination he is pale and has tachycardia. There is oozing of blood around the circumcision wound. A cannula is inserted and a blood cross-match sent. There is now oozing around the cannula site.

Investigation reveals:
- Hb (haemoglobin): 84 g/L
- WBC (white blood cell count): 12×10^9/L
- platelet count: 322×10^9/L
- prothrombin time: 16 seconds (control: 12–15 s)
- activated partial thromboplastin time: >120 seconds (control: 25–35 s)

23.7.2
Charlie, aged 5 years, is troubled by recurrent nose bleeds, the last of which took 1.5 hours to stop. He has no other medical problems. His examination is normal except for pale conjunctivae.

Investigation reveals:
- Hb (haemoglobin): 86 g/L
- WBC (white blood cells): 10.2×10^9/L
- platelet count: 350×10^9/L
- prothrombin time: 16 seconds (control: 12–15 s)
- activated partial thromboplastin time: 46 seconds (control: 25–35 s)
- fibrinogen: 2.5 g/L (normal: 2–4 g/L)
- factor VIII: just below the normal range

23.7.3
Melissa is a 3-year-old girl. She presents to her general practitioner with a 3–4 week history of lethargy and weight loss. On examination she is pale and has widespread bruising. She has no other medical history and is not currently on any medications.

The general practitioner orders a full blood count which reveals:
- Hb (haemoglobin): 66 g/L
- WBC (white blood cell): 43.2×10^9/L
- platelet count: 50×10^9/L

23.7.4
Xevera is a 7-year-old Greek boy who is seen by a paediatrician for constipation and was noted to look pale. Haematological testing reveals that he is anaemic with Hb of 100 g/L (both MCV and MCHC are low). He is given a course of iron therapy but his anaemia does not improve.

Further testing reveals 5% haemoglobin A_2 (HbA$_2$) and 3% fetal haemoglobin (HbF).

23.8
Below is a list (A–K) of treatment options. For each of the following patients with haematological problems select the appropriate treatment. Each option may be used once, more than once, or not at all.

A. Blood transfusion
B. Chemotherapy
C. Desmopressin
D. Folic acid supplementation
E. Intravenous antibiotics
F. Iron supplementation
G. No action required at present
H. Oral antibiotics
I. Recombinant factor VIII
J. Vitamin D
K. Vitamin K

23.8.1
Ahmed is a 4-week-old infant of Somali refugees who have just fled to the UK. He was circumcised yesterday, but the wound will not stop bleeding. On examination there is oozing of blood around the circumcision wound.

Investigation reveals:
- Hb (haemoglobin): 122 g/L
- WBC (white blood cell count): 11×10^9/L
- platelet count: 312×10^9/L
- prothrombin time: 36 seconds (control: 12–15 s)
- activated partial thromboplastin time: 25 seconds (control: 25–35 s)

23.8.2
Lola is an 8-month-old girl from Cyprus. She is referred to the paediatric department because she is clinically anaemic and has faltering growth. On examination you find that she has a large liver and spleen. Electrophoresis reveals an absence of haemoglobin A (HbA).

23.8.3
George is a 3-month-old boy. He presents to the paediatric ward with a swollen leg. He had an immunization yesterday and there is now a large swelling at the injection site. Haematological investigation reveals:
- Hb (haemoglobin): 102 g/L
- WBC (white blood cell count): 9.0×10^9/L
- platelet count: 312×10^9/L
- prothrombin time: 13 seconds (control: 12–15 s)
- activated partial thromboplastin time: 100 seconds (control: 25–35 s)

There is currently no bleeding and he is haemodynamically stable. His two older brothers both suffer from a bleeding disorder but both his parents and his older sister do not.

23.8.4

Lizzie is a 9-year-old girl who presents to the paediatric clinic. She is known to have hereditary spherocytosis. Her mother is concerned that she is very pale. Three weeks ago Lizzie had an upper respiratory tract infection. Her mother reports that she had a fever and was very flushed with bright red cheeks. She is otherwise well and has fully recovered from her infection. Her mother informs you that she has a very good diet. A full blood count reveals a Hb 88 g/L. A blood film reveals a normochromic normocytic anaemia with no blast cells.

23.8.5

Angie is 6 weeks old. She was jaundiced at 24 hours of age, when her haemoglobin (Hb) was checked and was 150 g/L. At 2 months of age she presents with an upper respiratory tract infection. The full blood count is repeated and she has Hb 102 g/L.

Answers: Single Best Answer

23.1
A. Acute lymphoblastic leukaemia
Acute lymphoblastic leukaemia is unlikely as she is well, has not had weight loss, and her splenomegaly is not accompanied by hepatomegaly or lymphadenopathy. Her blood count only shows anaemia, with normal white cell and platelet counts.

B. Glucose-6-phosphate dehydrogenase (G6PD) deficiency
G6PD deficiency may be associated with acute haemolysis but there would not usually be splenomegaly. In girls, clinical abnormalities are uncommon.

C. Hereditary spherocytosis ⊘
Correct. In hereditary spherocytosis the anaemia is usually mild (Hb 90–110 g/L), but the haemoglobin level may transiently fall during infections. Mild to moderate splenomegaly is common.

D. Sickle cell disease
Sickle cell disease would not be likely at all in a Caucasian child (see Fig. 23.12 in Illustrated Textbook of Paediatrics).

E. Thalassaemia
Thalassaemia is usually encountered in children from the Indian subcontinent, Mediterranean, and Middle East (see Fig. 23.12).

23.2
A. Acute lymphatic leukaemia
Acute lymphatic leukaemia is unlikely as he does not have abnormal clinical signs.

B. β-Thalassaemia trait
Thalassaemia trait patients rarely have symptoms but may be found to have anaemia.

C. Glucose-6-phosphate dehydrogenase deficiency ⊘
Correct. In G6PD deficiency, acute haemolysis may be precipitated by infection, the most common precipitating factor. Certain drugs including nitrofurantoin, fava beans (broad beans) and naphthalene in mothballs can also precipitate haemolysis. The urine is dark as it contains haemoglobin as well as urobilinogen.

D. Pyelonephritis
Pyelonephritis is unlikely as the child is afebrile and has no pain.

E. Sickle cell disease
Sickle cell disease is mostly seen in black children and adults.

23.3
A. Acute lymphoblastic leukaemia
In acute lymphoblastic leukaemia you would expect a range of abnormal clinical features.

B. Haemophilia A
In haemophilia A, thrombocytopenia is not a feature and the clotting profile would not be normal.

C. Immune thrombocytopenic purpura ⊘
Correct. Affected children develop petechiae, purpura, and/or superficial bruising. The platelet count can be very low (single digits) but treatment is not usually required and most cases resolve spontaneously.

D. Non-accidental injury
Non-accidental injury can present with unusual bruising but this boy has a low platelet count, which explains the bruising.

E. Vitamin D deficiency
In vitamin D deficiency, thrombocytopenia is not a feature.

23.4
A. Dietary advice
Dietary advice is required but iron therapy is a must as his anaemia is severe.

B. Folic acid
An important supplement for women prior to conception as it reduces the risk of neural tube defects in the fetus.

C. Iron supplements ⊘
Correct. Iron-deficiency anaemia is the most likely diagnosis and iron therapy is indicated. The presence of 'pica' strongly suggests iron deficiency. He may well be a picky eater and survives on cow's milk and little else.
In some children anaemia can be due to a β-thalassaemia trait. The blood parameters should be repeated after a course of treatment and if there has not been a response he should be tested for β-thalassaemia trait.

D. Multivitamin tablets
Vitamins are recommended for all preschool children but with such a significant anaemia and iron deficiency, a treatment course of iron is required first.

E. Vitamin B_{12} injections
A macrocytosis is usually seen in vitamin B_{12} deficiency, which is rare in children.

23.5
A. β-Thalassaemia trait
See Table 23.2 and Fig. 23.7 in Illustrated Textbook of Paediatrics. In β-thalassaemia trait, the haemoglobin A (HbA) would be approximately 90%. There would be extra fetal haemoglobin (HbF) and haemoglobin A_2 (HbA$_2$).

B. Glucose-6-phosphate dehydrogenase deficiency
Usually presents as either neonatal jaundice or acute haemolysis. Here the mean corpuscular

volume and the mean corpuscular haemoglobin are low suggesting a more chronic problem.

C. Iron-deficiency anaemia ⊘
Correct. A common diagnosis in children that results in these findings. The most common cause is dietary insufficiency (see Case History 23.1 in Illustrated Textbook of Paediatrics).

D. Normal variation for age and ethnicity
At 6 weeks of age children are in the 'physiological trough' for haemoglobin concentration and the lower limit of normal is 100 g/L. However, this is short lived and by 6 months, children maintain haemoglobin concentrations close to adult female levels. After puberty, boys have a higher normal range. See Fig. 23.2 in Illustrated Textbook of Paediatrics for more details.

E. Sickle cell trait
In sickle cell trait, there is inheritance of sickle haemoglobin (HbS) from one parent, so approximately 40% of the haemoglobin is HbS. Whilst carriers are asymptomatic, this is easily detectable on haemoglobin electrophoresis.

23.6
A. Acute lymphoblastic leukaemia
Although a small number of children present with bony pain, it would be unusual to have pain in the fingers.

B. β-Thalassaemia major
Would present with anaemia and if severe, this could lead to heart failure with peripheral oedema but pain would be unusual and there would be other signs. See Fig. 23.13 in Illustrated Textbook of Paediatrics for more details.

C. Glucose-6-phosphate dehydrogenase deficiency
After the neonatal period, this would present with acute haemolysis precipitated by infection, drugs or fava beans. Haemolysis is predominantly intravascular and is associated with fever, malaise and dark urine.

D. Haemophilia A
Haemophilia typically presents with bleeding into the larger joints.

E. Sickle cell disease ⊘
Correct. He is experiencing a vaso-occlusive crisis. A common clinical feature in late infancy is the hand–foot syndrome, in which there is dactylitis, with swelling and pain of the fingers and/or feet. His condition would be identified on the routine newborn screening blood test in the UK.

Answers: Extended Matching

Answer 23.7.1
H. Haemophilia A
Haemophilia usually presents with spontaneous bleeding into joints or muscles when infants

start to crawl or walk. However, it can present in the neonatal period with intracranial haemorrhage, bleeding after circumcision or prolonged oozing after heel sticks or venepuncture. The results of investigations in children with Haemophilia and von Willebrand disease are summarized in Table 23.3 in Illustrated Textbook of Paediatrics.

Answer 23.7.2
R. von Willebrand disease
On investigation, haemophilia A and von Willebrand disease (vWD) will both have a deranged activated partial thromboplastin time. However, in haemophilia A it is much more pronounced. The clinical features are also less pronounced in vWD, as in this child. Spontaneous soft-tissue bleeding, such as large haematomas, does not occur in vWD. A family history is common.

Answer 23.7.3
A. Acute lymphoblastic leukaemia
Lethargy, weight loss, bruising and anaemia, thrombocytopenia and raised white cell count suggest acute lymphoblastic leukaemia.

Answer 23.7.4
F. β-Thalassaemia trait
This boy most likely has a β-thalassaemia trait (see Table 23.2 in Illustrated Textbook of Paediatrics). A serum ferritin should have been performed prior to starting the iron therapy. This would most likely have been normal and iron therapy could have been avoided.

Answer 23.8.1
K. Vitamin K
This child probably has haemorrhagic disease of the newborn, due to vitamin K deficiency. In high-income countries prophylactic vitamin K is offered after birth. Vitamin K is essential for the production of active forms of factors II, VII, IX, and X and for the production of naturally occurring anticoagulants such as proteins C and S. Vitamin K deficiency therefore causes reduced levels of all of these factors. A clotting profile reveals a prolonged prothrombin time. He needs vitamin K treatment.

Answer 23.8.2
A. Blood transfusion
This girl has thalassaemia major. She will need life-long blood transfusions due to her profound anaemia. She will need iron chelation therapy to prevent the toxic effects of iron overload from excessive transfusions.

Answer 23.8.3
I. Recombinant factor VIII
In haemophilia A and von Willebrand disease there is an abnormal activated partial thromboplastin time and normal prothrombin time. However, in haemophilia A the abnormality

is far more pronounced. The family history also points towards haemophilia A, which is an X-linked recessive disorder. His factor VIII is low and treatment is needed.

Answer 23.8.4
G. No action required at present
She probably had a parvovirus infection associated with bone marrow suppression. This level of anaemia does not need transfusion. If she has a good diet, she will not need iron supplementation. However, she will need a further full blood count in a couple of weeks to ensure that her haemoglobin has not dropped further and reached the level where a blood transfusion is required. There is no absolute level below which transfusion is required but most children require blood when the haemoglobin is less than 50 g/L.

Answer 23.8.5
G. No action required at present
This is a normal variant. At birth, the haemoglobin in term infants is high, 140–215 g/L, to compensate for the low oxygen concentration in the fetus. The haemoglobin falls over the first few weeks, mainly due to reduced red cell production, reaching a nadir of around 100 g/L at 2 months of age (see Fig. 23.2 in Illustrated Textbook of Paediatrics).

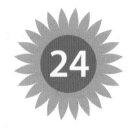

Child and adolescent mental health

Questions: Single Best Answer

24.1
James is a 3½-year-old boy who wets the bed about four of every seven nights. He does not wake after wetting. He has been dry during the day for 1 year. There is no history of constipation. He is otherwise well and has a normal examination. What would be the most appropriate initial management?

Select one answer only.

A. Desmopressin therapy
B. Enuresis alarm
C. 'Lifting' at midnight
D. Reassurance
E. Star chart

24.2
Zoe is a 14-year-old girl who has always been quiet and hard working. She is very thin and is losing weight despite being very interested in food; she enjoys baking cakes for her classmates and is always keen to go to the supermarket with her mother. Zoe herself denies that there is a problem with her weight or that she has been vomiting. Her parents are both extremely worried about her weight loss and poor appetite; they have not noticed any vomiting. There are no other symptoms and her examination is normal except that her height is on the 30th centile but her weight is below the 0.4th centile.

What is the most likely diagnosis?

Select one answer only.

A. Anorexia nervosa
B. Bulimia
C. Chronic fatigue syndrome
D. Coeliac disease
E. Depression

24.3
Florence is a 7-year-old girl whose mother brings her to her general practitioner. Her mother reports that Florence is hyperactive and that she is 'at the end of her tether'. Florence has always been a very active girl since learning to walk at 11 months of age. Although being described as an 'angel' at school, she is very difficult to manage at home. She is always on the go. She has tantrums when not getting her own way. She will often move from task to task at home without completing one before going on to the next. She has never been in any accidents and is not impulsive. Florence is currently staying with her grandparents two nights a week to give her mother a break. She has no other medical problems and is not on any medication. There is no family history of similar problems.

Which of the following would be the first step in management of this girl?

Select one answer only.

A. Parenting classes
B. Psychostimulant, e.g. methylphenidate
C. Referral to child psychiatrist
D. Referral to community paediatrician for specialist paediatric opinion
E. Sedative medication, e.g. sedating antihistamine

24.4
Georgio is a 6-year-old, normally healthy boy, who attends the Paediatric Assessment Unit. Three weeks ago he had a diarrhoeal illness lasting 3 days, which was not associated with vomiting and resolved without any treatment. Now he is having episodes of cramping abdominal pains. He has not opened his bowels for a week. He reports that his stools were normal prior to the diarrhoeal illness. He is his normal self between the episodes of abdominal pain. On examination he is a well child, not currently in pain, with an indentable mass in his left iliac fossa. His weight and height are plotted and are found to lie on the 25th centile.

What is the most likely diagnosis?

Select one answer only.

A. Appendicitis
B. Constipation
C. Intussusception
D. Malrotation with volvulus
E. Recurrent abdominal pain of childhood

24.5

Jeremy, aged 4 years, is brought to his general practitioner because he wakes some nights at about 10 pm with a shout. When his parents go to him he looks awake but confused. He goes back to sleep soon afterwards and next morning cannot recall any of these night-time events. He is otherwise well and has no medical problems.

What is the most likely explanation?

Select one answer only.

A. Complex partial seizures
B. Motor tics
C. Nightmares
D. Night terrors
E. Temper tantrums

24.6

For the last 3 months, Fatima, aged 13 years and born in the UK to parents of Pakistani origin, has complained of difficulty in doing school work, increased tiredness on the slightest exercise, pain in her joints and headaches with tenderness over the top of her head. This began shortly after a febrile illness, associated with a cough and sore throat, which lasted 3 days. She has not attended school for the last 8 weeks. Examination is normal. You plot her height and weight, which are on the 30th and 9th centile, respectively. There are no other medical problems and she is not on any medications.

On the basis of this history alone which of the following is the most likely diagnosis?

Select one answer only.

A. Chronic fatigue syndrome
B. Depression
C. Hypothyroidism
D. Juvenile dermatomyositis
E. Tuberculosis

24.7

Jane is 14 years old and has a diagnosis of chronic fatigue syndrome.

What would be the most appropriate management plan?

Select one answer only.

A. Complete bed rest
B. Gradual rehabilitation programme

C. Home tuition
D. Intensive exercise
E. Neurostimulant medication

Questions: Extended Matching

24.8

Below is a list (A–H) of possible interventions. For the scenarios described below, choose the most appropriate treatment interventions for emotional and behavioural problems in children and adolescents. Each option may be used once, more than once, or not at all.

A. Admit to paediatric ward
B. Cognitive behavioural therapy
C. Drug therapy
D. Explanation, advice and reassurance
E. Family therapy
F. Individual or group dynamic psychotherapy
G. Parenting group
H. Referral to a child psychiatrist

24.8.1

Steven is a 15-year-old boy who is brought to the Emergency Department. His mother is distressed because Steven is complaining that the television is putting thoughts into his head, and he is becoming increasingly suspicious of their next-door neighbour, who he believes is spying on him. His mood is normal and he is fully orientated. There is no suspicion of intoxication or medical cause for his symptoms. He has no other medical problems and is not on any medications.

24.8.2

Olivia is a 2-year-old girl who comes to the general paediatric clinic with her exasperated mother. Olivia throws tantrums whenever her mother asks her to do something that Olivia is reluctant to do. When you ask for an example, Olivia's mother describes breakfast time that morning, when Olivia screamed and threw her toast across the room when she was asked to stop flicking her yoghurt at her baby brother. Olivia was born at term and has no medical history.

24.8.3

Cynthia is a 15-year-old girl whose mother brings her to her general practitioner because of headaches and abdominal pain. These episodes of pain have been present for 6–9 months. There are no symptoms or signs to suggest an organic cause, so you ask some further questions. These reveal that Cynthia is bored most of the time, stays in her room and does not want to go out with her friends as she did previously. She used to be a star student, but now is doing less well in school. She often misses school because of feeling tired. She has no suicidal ideation and has never deliberately self-harmed. She is not on any medication.

Answers: Single Best Answer

24.1
A. Desmopressin therapy
This is likely to give short-term relief as desmopressin will stop the child making so much urine. Whilst this temporarily 'solves' the problem, it will not help him wake when his bladder becomes full. It is, however, very helpful for holidays or providing exhausted parents with some short-term relief. He is though too young to start this therapy.

B. Enuresis alarm
If an older child does not respond to a star chart, it may be supplemented with an enuresis alarm.

C. 'Lifting' at midnight
This might prevent the child waking with a wet bed but will not lead to any improvement in wakening.

D. Reassurance ⊘
Correct. Nocturnal enuresis is common at his age. About 6% of children aged 5 years and 3% of children aged 10 years have nocturnal enuresis.

E. Star chart
Probably the most effective treatment for most behavioural problems and most paediatricians would start using this around 5 years of age.

24.2
A. Anorexia nervosa ⊘
Correct. Zoe has several characteristic features – female, adolescent, weight below the 0.4th centile, but has a distorted body image in that she denies there is a problem with her weight. She has perfectionist personality traits and is overly interested in food without eating it herself.

B. Bulimia
Her parents do not think that she has been vomiting and so bulimia is less likely.

C. Chronic fatigue syndrome
There is no report of fatigue. Moreover, the weight loss and distorted body image are not usually symptoms of chronic fatigue syndrome.

D. Coeliac disease
Zoe denies that there is a problem with her weight. Although coeliac disease may (rarely) coexist, it does not fit well with the clinical history.

E. Depression
Features of depression are not present: she is not socially withdrawn and has enjoyment in life (e.g. baking cakes).

24.3
A. Parenting classes ⊘
Correct. Parenting classes are often effective in managing such problems. Many children are incorrectly labelled by family members or teachers as having attention deficit hyperactivity disorder. In this case her difficult behaviour is not pervasive, as it is not present at school.

B. Psychostimulant, e.g. methylphenidate
Although methylphenidate is a good treatment choice for moderately severe attention deficit hyperactivity disorder (ADHD), medication is reserved for those in whom behavioural interventions have been tried and failed. In the true *hyperkinetic disorder* or *ADHD*, the child is undoubtedly overactive in most situations (i.e. it is pervasive) and has impaired concentration with a short attention span or distractibility.

C. Referral to child psychiatrist
The symptoms described are common. Secondary care services would be overwhelmed if the first step is to refer all these children.

D. Referral to community paediatrician for specialist paediatric opinion
The symptoms described are common. Secondary care services would be overwhelmed if the first step is to refer all these children.

E. Sedative medication, e.g. sedating antihistamine
This would be unhelpful and would be likely to make things worse rather than better.

24.4
A. Appendicitis
There would be pain on abdominal examination. Classically, this would be in the right iliac fossa although a pelvic appendix can be more difficult to detect.

B. Constipation ⊘
Correct. The mass in his left iliac fossa is most likely to be impacted stool.

C. Intussusception
Intussusception causes intermittent abdominal pain, but has a shorter history, is usually found in younger children, and there would not be an indentable mass in the abdomen.

D. Malrotation with volvulus
Malrotation with volvulus may cause bilious vomiting and would not be associated with an indentable mass.

E. Recurrent abdominal pain of childhood
This is a common and important diagnosis but the presence of an indentable mass coupled with failure to open bowels for a week makes constipation more likely.

24.5
A. Complex partial seizures
Complex partial seizures do not present in this way. If the child wakes many times per night with episodes though, it is worth considering

rarer forms of seizure (nocturnal frontal lobe seizures).

B. Motor tics
Motor tics tend to be worse towards the end of the day (when the child is tired) or when watching/playing violent video games.

C. Nightmares
Nightmares usually occur later in the night or early morning as they occur most commonly during REM stages of sleep. They can usually be recalled.

D. Night terrors ⊘
Correct. Night terrors classically occur about 1–2 hours after falling asleep during the non-REM stage of sleep. The child is often confused, distressed and can appear terrified despite reassurances offered from parents. Unlike nightmares, there is no recollection of events the next day.

E. Temper tantrums
These do not wake a child from sleep. A child might have a tantrum upon being told to do something they do not want to.

24.6
A. Chronic fatigue syndrome ⊘
Correct. By definition, this is chronic fatigue syndrome. There are persisting high levels of subjective fatigue. Myalgia, migratory arthralgia and headaches are almost universal.

B. Depression
She does not report low mood or a lack of motivation.

C. Hypothyroidism
Some of the features described fit well with hypothyroidism but it is not the most likely cause. However, thyroid function tests form part of the investigations done in management of chronic fatigue syndrome.

D. Juvenile dermatomyositis
A rare diagnosis but one which can present with tiredness and muscle aches. The characteristic findings are an elevated creatinine kinase and a heliotrope rash across the eyelids.

E. Tuberculosis
No fevers and no family history of tuberculosis. It would be highly unusual for this to present in this way.

24.7
A. Complete bed rest
Complete bed rest can exacerbate the problem, leading to muscle atrophy and further fatigue.

B. Gradual rehabilitation programme ⊘
Correct. Usually the most successful approach in chronic fatigue syndrome. It consists of a gradual increase in exercise, school work and activities of daily living. Successful therapies include graded exercise tolerance programmes, pacing and cognitive behavioural therapy.

C. Home tuition
Home tuition can be useful but will not hasten recovery.

D. Intensive exercise
Intensive exercise can lead to relapse.

E. Neurostimulant medication
Neurostimulants have no place in management.

Answers: Extended Matching

Answer 24.8.1
H. Referral to a child psychiatrist
Steven has clinical features suggestive of schizophrenia, and needs a psychiatrist to assess him and manage his treatment.

Answer 24.8.2
D. Explanation, advice, and reassurance
This is a normal developmental stage, and needs advice about behaviour management.

Answer 24.8.3
B. Cognitive behavioural therapy
This may help her link feelings, thoughts and behaviour.

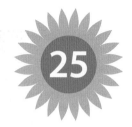

Dermatological disorders

Questions: Single Best Answer

25.1

William is a previously well 8-year-old boy who presents to the Emergency Department with a fever and arthralgia for 2 days, which is getting worse. On examination, he is noticed to have a painful, raised rash on his shins (Fig. 25.1).

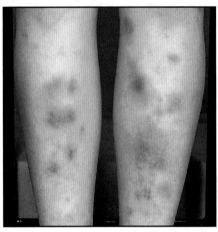

Figure 25.1 (Courtesy of Prof Julian Verbov)

Which of the following is the most likely cause?

Select one answer only.

A. Football injuries
B. Henoch–Schönlein purpura
C. Herpes simplex infection
D. *Mycoplasma pneumoniae* infection
E. Streptococcal infection

25.2

This 8-year-old boy presents to the Emergency Department. He is on co-trimoxazole (Septrin) as treatment for a urinary tract infection. He went on to develop severe ulceration of his mouth and corneal ulceration (Fig. 25.2).

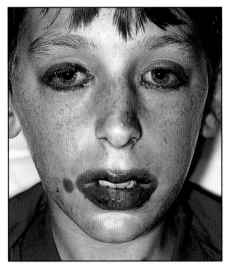

Figure 25.2 (Courtesy of Dr Rob Primhak)

What is the most likely diagnosis?

Select one answer only.

A. Kawasaki disease
B. Langerhans cell histiocytosis
C. Primary herpes simplex virus infection
D. Stevens–Johnson syndrome
E. Allergic keratoconjunctivitis

25.3

A 1-month-old male infant is brought to his family doctor. He has a rash confined to the perineum (Fig. 25.3). He has had diarrhoea for the last week.

What is the most likely cause for his rash?

Select one answer only.

A. Atopic eczema
B. *Candida* napkin rash
C. Chicken pox
D. Infantile seborrhoeic dermatitis
E. Irritant napkin rash

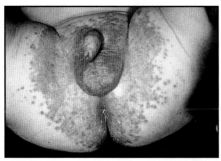

Figure 25.3 (Courtesy of Prof Julian Verbov)

25.4
Many rashes in childhood are itchy and can cause a lot of discomfort for the child.

Which of the following rashes is least likely to be itchy?

Select one answer only.

A. Atopic eczema
B. Chicken pox
C. Infantile seborrhoeic dermatitis
D. Pityriasis rosea
E. Scabies

25.5
You see William, a 10-month-old baby boy who has been diagnosed with atopic eczema. His parents are struggling to control it with herbal remedies. He is scratching himself all day and at night, and he appears in discomfort.

Which of the following is the most useful advice?

Select one answer only.

A. Apply emollients once a day
B. Bandages can only be used in children over 1 year of age
C. Regularly wash the baby with soap to avoid infection
D. Using nylon instead of cotton clothes
E. Use ointments instead of creams when the skin is dry

25.6
Mikey is a 2-year-old boy who has eczema. He comes to his family doctor with his mother, as his eczema has become troublesome over the last few weeks. His mother had been using emollients twice a day, but for the last few months during the summer she stopped as she did not think his eczema had been sufficiently bad. Today he has erythematous, weeping areas of skin in the flexor surfaces of his knees and ankles. There are also some areas of yellow crusting and he is pyrexial.

Which of the following is most likely to have caused his eczema to flare-up?

Select one answer only.

A. Bacterial infection
B. Exposure to allergen
C. Increase in heat due to summer
D. Reduction in his emollients
E. Viral infection

25.7
Robert is a 16-year-old boy with severe acne. He has had it for the last 3 years, but it is getting worse. He has tried some topical benzoyl benzoate sporadically but the skin lesions are now attracting adverse comments from his school friends, and he would like treatment. The lesions over his shoulder are shown (Fig. 25.4).

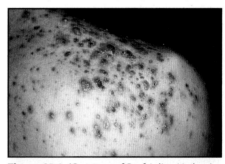

Figure 25.4 (Courtesy of Prof Julian Verbov)

What management would you recommend?

Select one answer only.

A. Continue with current regimen
B. Oral retinoid isotretinoin
C. Topical antibiotics
D. Topical benzoyl peroxide alone
E. Topical benzoyl peroxide and oral tetracycline

25.8
Joseph is a 4-year-old boy who is brought to the general paediatric clinic with this lesion in his hair (see Fig. 25.5 below).

What is the most likely diagnosis?

Select one answer only.

A. Alopecia areata
B. Cutis aplasia
C. Kerion
D. Langerhans cell histiocytosis
E. Psoriasis

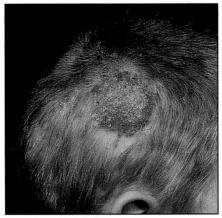

Figure 25.5 (Courtesy of Prof Julian Verbov)

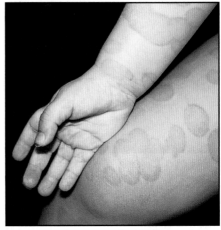

Figure 25.7 (Courtesy of Prof Julian Verbov)

25.9
Adam, a 2-day-old baby presents to the paediatric department as his mother is concerned about the appearance of his axilla, as shown in Fig. 25.6.

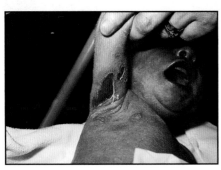

Figure 25.6

What is the cause of this?

Select one answer only.

A. Birth trauma
B. Burn
C. Eczema
D. Erythema toxicum
E. Infection

25.10
Stephan, a 5-year-old boy, presents with this rash (Fig. 25.7), which started 2 days ago. He had a mild fever, headache and cough for the last 5 days but is not particularly unwell. He was given amoxicillin by his general practitioner this morning and has taken one dose.

Which of the following is most likely to be the cause for the above rash?

A. Drug reaction
B. Inflammatory bowel disease
C. *Mycoplasma pneumoniae* infection
D. Tuberculosis
E. Varicella zoster

Questions: Extended Matching

25.11
For each of the following children select the most likely diagnosis (A–M). Each option may be used once, more than once, or not at all.

A. Acne vulgaris
B. Atopic eczema
C. Erythema multiforme
D. Guttate psoriasis
E. Henoch–Schönlein purpura
F. Immune thrombocytopenic purpura
G. Measles
H. Meningococcal disease
I. Molluscum contagiosum
J. Pityriasis rosea
K. Ringworm
L. Scabies
M. Systemic-onset juvenile idiopathic arthritis

25.11.1
Ashleigh is a 5-year-old girl. She presents to the Emergency Department with a non-blanching rash over her buttocks and legs (see Fig. 25.8 below). She is well in herself and has a heart rate of 100 beats/min, capillary refill of less than 2 seconds and is afebrile.

25.11.2
Edward, a 5-year-old boy presents to his general practitioner with a rash consisting of small

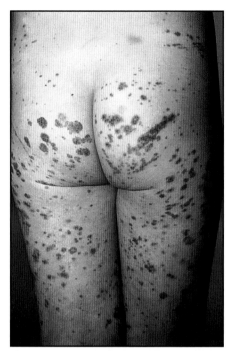

Figure 25.8

lesions which are erythematous and scaly on his trunks and limbs (Fig. 25.9). He has recently been diagnosed with a throat infection, but did not receive antibiotics.

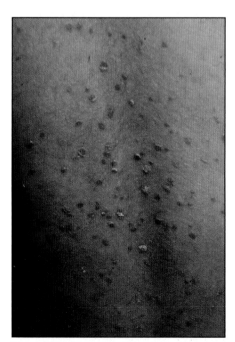

Figure 25.9 (Courtesy of Prof Julian Verbov)

25.11.3
A mother brings Noah, her 3-year-old son, to the general practitioner as she is concerned that her son's rash (Fig. 25.10) has been present for over 4 months.

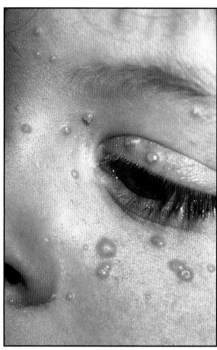

Figure 25.10 (Courtesy of Prof Julian Verbov)

25.11.4
Julie is a 10-month-old girl who has an intensely itchy rash on her hands, feet and wrists (Fig. 25.11).

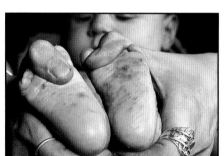

Figure 25.11

25.11.5
Damian is an 8-year-old boy. He has a persistent, itchy rash (see Fig. 25.12).

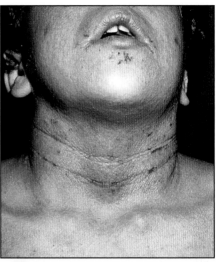

Figure 25.12 (Courtesy of Prof Julian Verbov)

Answers: Single Best Answer

25.1

A. Football injuries
Would be bruised. Why would he have
a fever?

B. Henoch–Schönlein purpura
Whilst joints are painful, the rash itself is not
painful and is purpuric and has a characteristic
distribution.

C. Herpes simplex infection
Herpes simplex can cause erythema
multiforme.

D. *Mycoplasma pneumoniae* infection
Mycoplasma pneumoniae can cause erythema
multiforme.

E. **Streptococcal infection** ⊘
Correct. This boy has erythema nodosum and the
causes include streptococcal infection, primary
tuberculosis, inflammatory bowel disease, drug
reaction or idiopathic.

25.2

A. Kawasaki disease
Kawasaki disease does cause a sore mouth and
bilateral non-purulent conjunctivitis. However, it
would not usually lead to ulceration. Fever
would be present for more than 5 days.

B. Langerhans cell histiocytosis
Langerhans cell histiocytosis is a rare diagnosis. It
sometimes is mistaken for eczema (see Fig. 22.19
in Illustrated Textbook of Paediatrics).

C. Primary herpes simplex virus infection
The rash shown does not have the vesicular
pattern typically seen with herpes simplex virus
infection (HSV), nor the characteristic clinical
features.

D. **Stevens–Johnson syndrome** ⊘
Correct. This boy has Stevens–Johnson
syndrome, which is a severe bullous form of
erythema multiforme. Its relative frequency in
children treated with co-trimoxazole has led
to this antibiotic rarely being used. It is still
helpful for the treatment or prevention of
Pneumocystis jirovecii (*carinii*) in children with
immunosuppression. The eye involvement may
include conjunctivitis, corneal ulceration and
uveitis, and ophthalmological assessment is
required. It may also be caused by sensitivity to
other drugs or infection, with morbidity and
sometimes even mortality from infection,
toxaemia or renal damage.

E. Allergic keratoconjunctivitis
Severe allergy can be very unpleasant but would
not cause this severity of conjunctivitis or lip/
mouth involvement.

25.3

A. Atopic eczema
Atopic eczema is rarely present at this age, and
appears predominantly on the face and trunk of
infants.

B. *Candida* **napkin rash** ⊘
Correct. In this condition the flexures are
involved and there are satellite lesions (isolated
erythematous lesions away from the main
rash area).

C. Chicken pox
Chicken pox is a vesicular rash.

D. Infantile seborrhoeic dermatitis
Infantile seborrhoeic dermatitis is more discrete
than this rash, which is widespread.

E. Irritant napkin rash
In irritant napkin rash the flexures are spared.

25.4

A. Atopic eczema
A key feature of eczema is itch. This
causes the child to scratch, which exacerbates
the condition and predisposes to local
infection.

B. Chicken pox
This is very itchy, particularly in the healing phase.
Scratching can lead to permanent scarring and is
often treated with calamine lotion.

C. **Infantile seborrhoeic dermatitis** ⊘
Correct. The causes of itchy rashes are: atopic
eczema, chicken pox, urticaria, allergic reactions,
contact dermatitis, insect bites, scabies, fungal
infections and pityriasis rosea.
All the conditions listed in the question are itchy
other than seborrhoeic dermatitis.

D. Pityriasis rosea
A typical feature is itch.

E. Scabies
If the itch is shared, then always consider
scabies. Indeed, it is a truism in dermatology
that any persistent itchy rash should be
considered as scabies until this has been
excluded.

25.5

A. Apply emollients once a day
There are many different management
options for eczema. Simple advice includes
using emollients frequently – at least twice
a day, but do not use sparingly. A typical
infant will use 250–500 ml of emollient every
fortnight.

B. Bandages can only be used in children over 1
year of age
Occlusive bandages are extremely helpful at
any age, especially when excoriation and
lichenification are a problem.

C. Regularly wash the baby with soap to avoid infection
There are many different management options for eczema. Simple advice includes avoiding soap.

D. Using nylon instead of cotton clothes
Avoiding nylon and woollen clothes is useful.

E. Use ointments instead of creams when the skin is dry ⊘
Correct. Ointments are preferable to creams when the skin is dry.

25.6
A. Bacterial infection ⊘
Correct. Causes of flare-up of eczema are:
- bacterial infection, e.g. *Staphylococcus*, *Streptococcus* spp.
- viral infection, e.g. herpes simplex virus
- ingestion of an allergen, e.g. egg
- contact with an irritant or allergen
- environment: heat, humidity
- change or reduction in medication
- psychological stress.

The yellow crusting and pyrexia are suggestive of infection with *Staphylococcus*, therefore a bacterial cause for the exacerbation.

B. Exposure to allergen
But why would he be pyrexial?

C. Increase in heat due to summer
Would this cause the crusting?

D. Reduction in his emollients
A cause but why would there be weeping? A weeping skin should prompt one to start antibiotics.

E. Viral infection
If it was vesicular, then always consider herpes simplex. If he is ill enough to warrant hospital admission, then antivirals are often given in conjunction with antibiotics whilst awaiting improvement.

25.7
A. Continue with current regimen
It is not working.

B. Oral retinoid isotretinoin
Oral retinoid isotretinoin is reserved for severe acne that is unresponsive to other treatments.

C. Topical antibiotics
Topical antibiotics and sunshine can be helpful but probably only in milder disease and this is severe.

D. Topical benzoyl peroxide alone
Benzoyl peroxide on its own will probably not be adequate.

E. Topical benzoyl peroxide and oral tetracycline ⊘
Correct. Robert has severe acne with marked cystic and nodular lesions. Benzoyl peroxide will need to be combined with oral antibiotics.

25.8
A. Alopecia areata
Usually flat, colourless, and painless. Not swollen and red.

B. Cutis aplasia
A scalp defect that presents at birth.

C. Kerion ⊘
Correct. Kerions are caused by infection with tinea capitis (scalp ringworm). Topical treatment is usually tried first but oral antifungals may be required for very severe cases.

D. Langerhans cell histiocytosis
Causes a seborrhoeic rash in infants. It is rare.

E. Psoriasis
The rash shown is localized and not scaly as in psoriasis.

25.9
A. Birth trauma
There would be bruising and this site would be highly unusual with birth trauma.

B. Burn
A burn in that distribution and no history is very unlikely.

C. Eczema
Eczema does not cause blistering and the infant is too young.

D. Erythema toxicum
Erythema toxicum is a benign pustular rash that migrates and requires no treatment.

E. Infection ⊘
Correct. Staphylococcal infection causing blistering. There are several variations of this from bullous impetigo to staphylococcal scalded skin syndrome, as shown here.

25.10
A. Drug reaction
This is a possible cause, but here the rash preceded the first dose of antibiotic.

B. Inflammatory bowel disease
Inflammatory bowel disease is associated with erythema nodosum.

C. *Mycoplasma pneumonia* infection ⊘
Correct. The rash is erythema multiforme. Although amoxicillin can cause this rash, it was given after the rash appeared. Other causes of erythema multiforme include herpes simplex virus or idiopathic. His symptoms are consistent with *Mycoplasma pneumoniae* infection.

D. Tuberculosis
A cause of erythema multiforme but unlikely with this history.

E. Varicella zoster
Varicella zoster virus causes a vesicular rash.

Answers: Extended Matching

Answer 25.11.1
E. Henoch–Schönlein purpura
The rash here is typical of Henoch–Schönlein purpura. A classic triad of colicky abdominal pain, arthralgia and purpuric rash often develop, but in the early stages the rash usually predominates.

Answer 25.11.2
D. Guttate psoriasis
The presentation here is typical and often a flare of guttate psoriasis follows an infection. Scaly rashes should always raise the possibility of psoriasis.

Answer 25.11.3
I. Molluscum contagiosum
This is caused by a poxvirus. The lesions are small, skin-coloured, pearly papules with central umbilication. They may be single but are usually multiple. Lesions are often widespread but tend to disappear spontaneously within a year.

Answer 25.11.4
L. Scabies
Always consider scabies if a rash is very itchy. It is a highly contagious (and unpleasant) condition.

Answer 25.11.5
B. Atopic eczema
Atopic eczema affects 20% of children. Lichenification and erythema are shown. The skin looks sore and the excoriations suggest itch. The face often remains affected from undue reluctance to use topical steroids on the face of a child of this age.

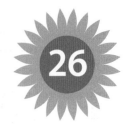

Diabetes and endocrinology

Questions: Single Best Answer

26.1

Ellie, a 7-year-old girl, is newly diagnosed with diabetes mellitus. She has been drinking lots of fluid and has had to pass urine frequently. She has a markedly raised blood glucose (20 mmol/L) and heavy glycosuria.

Which of the following is most likely to be true about her diabetes?

Select one answer only.

A. Her diagnosis should be confirmed with an oral glucose tolerance test
B. She can be managed with oral hypoglycaemic agents and dietary modification
C. She will have gained weight in the last few weeks
D. The incidence in the UK is falling
E. There is autoimmune pancreatic β-cell damage

26.2

James, aged 11 years, has type 1 diabetes mellitus. While playing football during the mid-morning break at a holiday camp, he suddenly feels faint. His classmates call the supervisor who finds him lying unresponsive in the playground.

What should be his immediate management?

Select one answer only.

A. Call an ambulance
B. Check blood glucose
C. Give a glucose drink
D. Give buccal glucose gel
E. Give insulin

26.3

Catherine, aged 15 years, has had type 1 diabetes mellitus for 7 years. Her insulin regimen has remained unchanged for the last 7 months. Her HbA$_{1c}$ has increased from 58 mmol/mol (7.5%) to 90 mmol/mol (10.3%) (desired level <58 mmol/mol). The most recent blood glucose levels as recorded in her book are shown in Fig. 26.1 (overleaf):

What is the most likely explanation for these findings?

Select one answer only.

A. During the summer holidays she took less exercise
B. She has reduced her insulin dosage to try to lose weight
C. She is taking more insulin than she needs
D. She is regularly eating snacks and indulging in high carbohydrate food
E. Some of the blood glucose measurements are fictitious

26.4

Mohammed, a 12-year-old boy with type 1 diabetes mellitus, is reviewed in the outpatient clinic. In spite of maintaining good control of his diabetes, his height has remained static for 9 months. He says his appetite is alright, but he has lost interest in football, which is his passion, as he says he can't keep up with the other boys any more. He just stays at home and watches TV, but wants to be out playing football and getting back his energy. A full blood count and C-reactive protein are normal and his HbA$_{1c}$ is satisfactory.

What is the most likely diagnosis?

Select one answer only.

A. Anorexia nervosa
B. Depression
C. Growth hormone deficiency
D. Hypothyroidism
E. Inflammatory bowel disease

Please refer to your Doctor or Diabetes Nurse specialist as to when you should perform your tests.

Date	Insulin injection (Time / Dosage)				Blood: Before breakfast	Blood: 2hr after breakfast	Blood: Before mid-day meal	Blood: 2hr after mid-day meal	Blood: Before evening meal	Blood: 2hr after evening meal	Blood: Before bed	Blood: During night	Comments
21/9							4						
22/9									4				
23/9								8					
24/9							5						
25/9													Visiting nan
26/9					5								
27/9										4			
28/9							4						
29/9						8							
30/9									10				
1/10											4		
2/10													Visiting nan
3/10								4					
4/10									3				
5/10								9					
6/10										8			
7/10						6							
8/10							4						
9/10									4				
10/10											6		
11/10											7		
12/10							5						

Figure 26.1

26.5

Zeinab, aged 15 years, has had 3 months of diarrhoea, weight loss and palpitations. You suspect hyperthyroidism.

Which combination of thyroid function test results would confirm the diagnosis?

Select one answer only.

A. High TSH and high T_4 levels
B. High TSH and low T_4 levels
C. Low TSH and high T_4 levels
D. Low TSH and low T_4 levels
E. Normal TSH and high T_4 levels

26.6

Lara, an 18-day-old female infant, has congenital adrenal hypoplasia. She presents having vomited all her feeds today. She has become lethargic and will no longer feed. On examination she has tachycardia, with a heart rate of 160 beats/min and a capillary refill time of 3 seconds. A bedside blood test shows that she is hypoglycaemic.

What is the best immediate management?

Select one answer only.

A. Intravenous glucose alone for 24 hours
B. Intravenous saline, glucose and hydrocortisone
C. Oral rehydration
D. Oral rehydration and oral glucocorticoid
E. Oral rehydration, sodium supplements and oral glucocorticoid

26.7

Amy, aged 8 years, is rapidly putting on weight. A photograph of her is shown in Fig. 26.2. She has truncal obesity and striae on her abdomen.

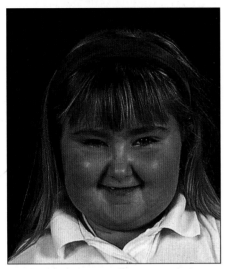

Figure 26.2 (Courtesy of Dr Jerry Wales)

What is the most likely cause for this?

Select one answer only.

A. Corticosteroid cream for severe eczema
B. Daily oral prednisolone therapy for the last 6 months
C. Ectopic ACTH (adrenocorticotropic hormone)-producing tumour
D. High-dose corticosteroid therapy for lung disease when she was a premature baby
E. Long-term use of inhaled corticosteroids

26.8

Luke, a 4-month-old male infant, presents with a history of vomiting and diarrhoea. On examination he has a heart rate of 160 beats/min; his capillary refill time is 2–3 seconds and he is lethargic. A bedside blood test showed that he is hypoglycaemic. A diagnosis of Addison disease is considered.

Which of the following combination of biochemical results would be most likely with Addison's disease?

Select one answer only.

A. Hypernatraemia and hyperkalaemia with low cortisol
B. Hypernatraemia and hypokalaemia with high cortisol
C. Hyponatraemia and hyperkalaemia with high cortisol
D. Hyponatraemia and hypokalaemia with low cortisol
E. Hyponatraemia and hyperkalaemia with low cortisol

26.9

George, a 2-week-old male infant, presents to the Emergency Department with vomiting, diarrhoea and poor feeding.

Investigations show:

- sodium 112 mmol/L (normal range 133–145 mmol/L)
- potassium 6.8 mmol/L (normal range 3.5–6.0 mmol/L)
- urea 7.8 mmol/L (normal range 2.5–8.0 mmol/L)
- creatinine 30 mmol/L (normal range 20–65 mmol/L)
- blood glucose 1.7 mmol/L (normal range >2.6 mmol/L)
- infection screen—negative

What is the most likely cause?

Select one answer only.

A. Acute kidney injury
B. Congenital adrenal hyperplasia
C. Congenital adrenal hypoplasia
D. Cushing syndrome
E. Gastroenteritis

26.10

A newborn baby has recently been delivered. The midwife requests an urgent paediatric review of the baby because she cannot tell if the baby is male or female (Fig. 26.3). The parents are asking what sex their baby is.

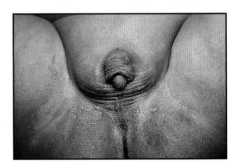

Figure 26.3

What should you tell them?

Select one answer only.

A. You are unable to tell if the baby is male or female, and tell the parents it is likely to be a mixture of both sexes, i.e. ovotesticular disorder of sex development (DSD – or hermaphroditism)
B. You are unable to tell right now and a detailed assessment of the baby including scans and blood tests will be needed before a specialist can tell them

C. You are unable to tell right now but will be able to assign a sex as soon as you get the baby's chromosomes back
D. You think it is likely to be a girl so tell them the baby should be named as a female on the birth certificate pending the results
E. You think it is likely to be a boy so tell them the child should be named as a male on the birth certificate pending the results

26.11

A baby is born with a disorder of sexual differentiation. Congenital adrenal hyperplasia is suspected.

What blood result would confirm the diagnosis?

Select one answer only.

A. A low testosterone
B. A markedly lowered plasma 17 α–hydroxyprogesterone
C. A markedly raised cortisol level
D. A markedly raised plasma 17α-hydroxyprogesterone
E. A raised blood glucose

Questions: Extended Matching

26.12

For each of the following scenarios chose the best course of action (A–K) to take immediately.

A. Buccal glucose gel
B. Diet therapy alone
C. Fluid resuscitation with normal saline (0.9% sodium chloride)
D. Insulin infusion intravenously
E. Intramuscular (IM) glucagon
F. Intravenous antibiotics
G. Intravenous infusion of 5% glucose
H. Intravenous infusion of normal saline (0.9% sodium chloride)
I. Intravenous sodium bicarbonate
J. Oral glucose drink
K. Subcutaneous insulin

26.12.1

Julie, aged 7 years, has diabetes mellitus. She is admitted to hospital as she has vomited on three occasions. She has a 2-day history of being unwell with a mild fever, sore throat and decreased appetite. Her blood glucose measurement reads 'high'. Although she was not eating, her parents maintained her usual insulin dose. On examination her temperature is 37.5°C. She is drowsy and confused. Her pulse is 150 beats/min, blood pressure 80/45 mmHg (low for age) and capillary refill time 3 seconds. Examination of her throat shows tonsillitis. Her blood glucose is 22 mmol/L.

26.12.2

Jon is 12 years old. His brother has diabetes. He has started to drink a lot of fluids and pass a lot of urine. He checked his blood glucose on his brother's glucometer. It was 19 mmol/L. When he arrives in the Emergency Department he is well with no signs of dehydration. Diabetes mellitus type 1 is diagnosed as his blood glucose is 21 mmol/L. A venous blood sample shows a normal pH with 2 mmol/L of ketones (within the normal range) and a HbA1c blood test result is awaited.

26.12.3

Harriet, a 5-year-old girl, is known to have diabetes mellitus type 1. She was only diagnosed 2 months ago and is on a basal bolus regime of insulin. She is running around the garden at home when her mother notices she suddenly becomes aggressive towards her brother and looks pale and not her usual self. Her mother checks her blood glucose, which is 3 mmol/L.

26.12.4

Sophie, a 9-year-old girl with type 1 diabetes mellitus, develops a fever along with vomiting and diarrhoea. After 2 days her mother takes her to the local paediatric assessment unit as she continues to vomit. On examination her temperature is 37.5°C. She is able to talk to her mother. She has clinical dehydration. Her pulses, capillary refill time and blood pressure are normal. Her blood glucose is 16 mmol/L.

Answers: Single Best Answer

26.1
A. Her diagnosis should be confirmed with an oral glucose tolerance test
An oral glucose tolerance test is not required as her clinical presentation and investigations have established the diagnosis. The test is seldom required to diagnose diabetes in children, though it may be used to screen for cystic fibrosis related diabetes mellitus.

B. She can be managed with oral hypoglycaemic agents and dietary modification
She requires insulin.

C. She will have gained weight in the last few weeks
Weight loss is a feature at presentation.

D. The incidence in the UK is falling
She has type 1 diabetes mellitus. In the UK its incidence is increasing and now affects 2 per 1000 children under 16 years of age.

E. There is autoimmune pancreatic β-cell damage ⊘
Correct. Almost all (>95%) children in the UK have type 1 diabetes mellitus which occurs as a result of autoimmune destruction of pancreatic β-cells by T cells.

26.2
A. Call an ambulance
This will be required if he does not respond to initial treatment. The holiday camp should be prepared for treatment of hypoglycaemia in a known diabetic.

B. Check blood glucose
He has the clinical features of hypoglycaemia and immediate treatment is indicated.

C. Give a glucose drink
This is appropriate if he can take fluids, but he is unresponsive.

D. Give buccal glucose gel ⊘
Correct. He is hypoglycaemic, brought on by exercise. Glucose is absorbed quickly from buccal glucose gel, and he should rapidly wake up. He will need to have a carbohydrate-containing drink and snack to maintain his blood glucose.

E. Give insulin
His blood glucose needs to be raised rather than lowered.

26.3
A. During the summer holidays she took less exercise
She would be expected to have had more exercise over the summer holidays.

B. She has reduced her insulin dosage to try to lose weight
Reducing the insulin dose would result in high blood glucose levels and not the normal values shown in the diary.

C. She is taking more insulin than she needs
More insulin than she needs would result in low blood glucose levels and the HbA$_{1C}$ would not have increased.

D. She is regularly eating snacks and indulging in high carbohydrate food
Regularly eating snacks and indulging in high carbohydrate food would result in high blood glucose levels and not the normal values shown in the diary.

E. Some of the blood glucose measurements are fictitious ⊘
Correct. Some of the blood glucose measurements are fictitious. Most of the values recorded are normal but her diabetic control has deteriorated and is no longer in the desired range.

26.4
Anorexia nervosa
Eating disorders can co-exist with diabetes mellitus but he does not have the clinical features of anorexia nervosa.

B. Depression
Depression is also important to consider, but in this case, it is not the most likely cause as he is continuing to maintain good control of his diabetes and is not expressing negative feelings.

C. Growth hormone deficiency
Not an autoimmune problem. Would not explain his lethargy.

D. Hypothyroidism ⊘
Correct. Children with type 1 diabetes mellitus are at increased risk of thyroid disease and should be screened annually. His static height and his lethargy would support this diagnosis. He is also at increased risk of coeliac disease and this should also be considered but is less likely as his appetite is good and his weight is satsifactory.

E. Inflammatory bowel disease
Blood and mucus in the stool would be expected with ulcerative colitis and anorexia and malaise and abnormal full blood count and C-reactive protein would be expected with Crohn's disease.

26.5
A. High TSH and high T$_4$ levels
Central cause for hyperthyroidism would be very rare.

B. High TSH and low T$_4$ levels
Suggests that thyroid gland is not working. Would result in hypothyroidism.

C. Low TSH and high T₄ levels ⊘

Correct. Hyperthyroidism usually results from autoimmune thyroiditis (Graves disease) secondary to the production of thyroid-stimulating immunoglobulins (TSIs). The levels of thyroxine (T_4) and/or tri-iodothyronine (T_3) are elevated and TSH levels are suppressed to very low levels.

D. Low TSH and Low T₄ levels
Central hypothyroidism.

E. Normal TSH and high T₄ levels
Very early change. Would soon be followed by a fall in TSH.

26.6
A. Intravenous glucose alone for 24 hours
No. The child is having a salt-losing crisis.

B. Intravenous saline, glucose and hydrocortisone ⊘
Correct. Lara is having an adrenal crisis. This requires urgent treatment with intravenous saline, glucose and hydrocortisone. Long-term treatment is with glucocorticoid and mineralocorticoid replacement and oral sodium chloride may be needed during infancy. The dose of glucocorticoid needs to be increased at times of illness.

C. Oral rehydration
Always helpful but in this case not sufficient treatment.

D. Oral rehydration and oral glucocorticoid
This child is seriously ill. There isn't time to lose.

E. Oral rehydration, sodium supplements and oral glucocorticoid
All the correct things are being replaced here but this is an emergency and it requires more rapid correction.

26.7
A. Corticosteroid cream for severe eczema
Topical steroids do not cause this because the doses absorbed systemically are low.

B. Daily oral prednisolone therapy for the last 6 months ⊘
Correct. Children requiring high dose oral corticosteroid therapy, e.g. for Crohn's disease or nephrotic syndrome, may develop the features of Cushing syndrome. Minimized by decreasing the dose as soon as possible.

C. Ectopic ACTH (adrenocorticotropic hormone)-producing tumour
Extremely rare in children. However, must be considered if there is no history of steroid use.

D. High-dose corticosteroid therapy for lung disease when she was a premature baby
A short course of steroids in the premature period, even if high-dose, would not cause features of Cushing syndrome at this age.

E. Long-term use of inhaled corticosteroids
She has Cushing syndrome. Inhaled steroids are unlikely to cause this because the doses absorbed systemically are low.

26.8
A. Hypernatraemia and hyperkalaemia with low cortisol
The laboratory findings in Addison disease are low sodium.

B. Hypernatraemia and hypokalaemia with high cortisol
Wrong way around.

C. Hyponatraemia and hyperkalaemia with high cortisol
The cortisol level would be low.

D. Hyponatraemia and hypokalaemia with low cortisol
The potassium is typically high.

E. Hyponatraemia and hyperkalaemia with low cortisol ⊘
Correct. In Addison disease, there is hyponatraemia, hyperkalaemia and hypoglycaemia. The plasma cortisol is low and the plasma ACTH (adrenocorticotropic hormone) concentration is high. See Box 26.10 in Illustrated Textbook of Paediatrcs for more details.

26.9
A. Acute kidney injury
Hyponatraemia may be a feature of acute kidney injury, but this child has a normal plasma urea and creatinine.

B. Congenital adrenal hyperplasia ⊘
Correct. The combination of marked hyponatraemia, hyperkalaemia and hypoglycaemia are suggestive of glucocorticoid deficiency, as seen in congenital adrenal hyperplasia.

C. Congenital adrenal hypoplasia
Much rarer than congenital adrenal hyperplasia but also can result in hyponatremia, hyperkalaemia and hypoglycaemia. There are X-linked (early onset) and autosomal recessive (variable onset) forms.

D. Cushing syndrome
An excess of glucocorticoids, as seen in Cushing syndrome, causes an intolerance to carbohydrates (hyperglycaemia), rather than the hypoglycaemia seen in this child.

E. Gastroenteritis
Gastroenteritis can lead to hyponatraemic dehydration, but the urea would be raised and the potassium normal.

26.10
A. You are unable to tell if the baby is male or female, and tell the parents it is likely to be a mixture of both sexes, i.e. ovotesticular disorder of sex development (DSD – or hermaphroditism)

This is extremely rare. It is usually possible to assign the infant a sex after assessment of phenotype, sex hormones and ultrasound scans of internal structures and gonads are performed.

B. You are unable to tell right now and a detailed assessment of the baby including scans and blood tests will be needed before a specialist can tell them ⊘
Correct. A detailed assessment by medical, surgical and psychological specialists needs to be performed followed by a full discussion with the parents before the infant is assigned a sex.

C. You are unable to tell right now but will be able to assign a sex as soon as you get the baby's chromosomes back
Sexuality is complex, and depends on more than the baby's phenotype, chromosomes and hormone levels.

D. You think it is likely to be a girl so tell them the baby should be named as a female on the birth certificate pending the results
If there is abnormal sexual differentiation at birth, do not guess the infant's gender. A detailed assessment needs to be performed.

E. You think it is likely to be a boy so tell them the child must be named as a male on the birth certificate pending the results
If there is abnormal sexual differentiation at birth, do not guess the infant's gender. A detailed assessment needs to be performed.

26.11
A. A low testosterone
In congenital adrenal hyperplasia the testosterone would be raised.

B. A markedly lowered plasma 17 α–hydroxyprogesterone
In most cases, the 17 α–hydroxyprogesterone is markedly raised. You might see this in the much less common congenital adrenal hypoplasia though.

C. A markedly raised cortisol level
In congenital adrenal hyperplasia the cortisol level would be low.

D. A markedly raised plasma 17α-hydroxyprogesterone ⊘
Most children with congenital adrenal hyperplasia have 21-hydroxylase deficiency (see Fig. 26.11 in Illustrated Textbook of Paediatrics). The diagnosis is made by finding markedly raised levels of the metabolic precursor 17 α-hydroxy-progesterone.

E. A raised blood glucose
It would typically be low.

Answers: Extended Matching

Answer 26.12.1
C. Fluid resuscitation with normal saline (0.9% sodium chloride)
Julie requires immediate fluid resuscitation as she has diabetic ketoacidosis and is in shock. See Fig. 26.7a, Illustrated Textbook of Paediatrics.

Answer 26.12.2
K. Subcutaneous insulin
Start insulin subcutaneously. Although this is a new diagnosis of diabetes of mellitus, Jon is well so it is safe to start subcutaneous insulin. He also requires education about diabetes, changes to diet and lifestyle, training on how to administer the insulin, and what to do in an emergency.

Answer 26.12.3
J. Oral glucose drink
Harriet is hypoglycaemic and requires some sugar to increase her blood glucose. The easiest way to achieve this is with a non-diet sugary drink. She will require complex carbohydrate snacks to maintain her blood glucose.

Answer 26.12.4
H. Intravenous infusion of normal saline (0.9% sodium chloride)
Intravenous 0.9% sodium chloride solution is required, as she continues to vomit and has clinical dehydration. She does not require fluid resuscitation as she is not shocked.

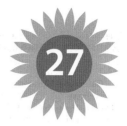
Inborn errors of metabolism

27.1
A newborn baby is diagnosed with a metabolic condition at 10 days of age, after she presented with vomiting, jaundice, hepatomegaly and liver failure. She was subsequently put on a lactose-free and galactose-free diet.

Which enzyme is most likely to be deficient?

Select one answer only.

A. Galactokinase
B. Galactose-1-phosphate uridyl transferase
C. Glucose-6-phosphatase
D. Glucose-6- phosphate dehydrogenase
E. Phosphoglucomutase

27.2
Samina is 12-years-old and has hepatomegaly. She is short for her age, suffers from hypoglycaemia and needs an overnight feed via a nasogastric tube.

What is the most likely diagnosis?

Select one answer only.

A. Congenital adrenal hyperplasia
B. Familial hypercholesterolaemia
C. Glycogen storage disorder
D. Phenylketonuria
E. Urea cycle defect

27.3
Terry was born at term and was well at birth. On day 2 of life, he became severely unwell with poor feeding, vomiting, acidosis and encephalopathy. Sepsis and hypoglycaemia were excluded, and an inborn error of metabolism is thought to be the cause as the blood ammonia level is extremely high. Which of the following is the most likely cause?

Select one answer only.

A. Fatty acid oxidation defect
B. Glycogen storage disease
C. MCAD (Medium-chain acyl-CoA dehydrogenase deficiency)
D. Mucopolysaccharidosis
E. Urea cycle defect

Answers: Single Best Answer

27.1
B. Galactose-1-phosphate uridyl transferase ⊘

Correct. The baby has been put on a diet that excludes galactose. The enzyme defect is therefore likely to be one involving galactose. This infant has galactosaemia, which is a rare disorder resulting from deficiency of the enzyme galactose-1-phosphate uridyl transferase, which is essential for galactose metabolism. When lactose-containing milk feeds such as breast milk or infant formula are introduced, affected infants feed poorly, vomit, develop jaundice, hepatomegaly and hepatic failure. Management is with a lactose-free and galactose-free diet for life.

27.2
C. Glycogen storage disorder ⊘

Correct. She has clinical features of the hepatic form of glycogen storage disorder, where enzyme defects prevent the mobilization of glucose from glycogen and gluconeogenesis, resulting in abnormal storage of glycogen in liver.

27.3
A. Fatty acid oxidation defect
These disorders, e.g. carnitine transporter deficiency, may present in an infant or older child with an illness similar to this but with hypoglycaemia as a prominent feature and the blood ammonia level may be raised but not to extremely high levels. May also present as an acute life-threatening episode (ALTE) or near-miss sudden infant death syndrome (SIDS).

B. Glycogen storage disease
Enzyme defects prevent glycogen synthesis or breakdown in liver and/or muscle. Liver forms present with severe hypoglycaemia and hepatomegaly; muscle forms with exercise intolerance.

C. MCAD (Medium-chain acyl-CoA dehydrogenase deficiency)
Detected on neonatal biochemical screening, or presents with acute encephalopathy and hypoglycaemia on fasting, or as an acute life-threatening episode (ALTE) or near-miss sudden infant death syndrome (SIDS). Acute illness may sometimes develop before screening results are known.

D. Mucopolysaccharidosis
After a period of normal development development regresses, facies become coarse and organomegaly develops. Skeletal abnormalities are relatively common, particularly of the ribs and vertebrae.

E. Urea cycle defect ⊘

Correct. Urea cycle or organic acid disorders may present with these clinical features. The marked hyperammonaemia is characteristic of urea cycle defects.

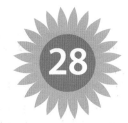
Musculoskeletal disorders

Questions: Single Best Answer

28.1

Amir is a 5-year-old boy who was born and lives in the UK. His parents are from Pakistan. He presents to the Emergency Department with a high temperature and complains of pain in his right upper arm. This has been present for 2 days and seems to be getting worse. The pain is described as being sharp and gets worse when he moves his arm. He had an abscess on his right finger 2 weeks ago for which he was prescribed oral antibiotics. On examination he has a temperature of 39°C. There is an area of redness and swelling over the right upper arm which is painful when touched or moved. The white cell count and C-reactive protein level are raised.

What is the most likely causative organism of his infection?

Select one answer only.

A. *Haemophilus influenzae*
B. *Mycobacterium tuberculosis*
C. *Salmonella typhi*
D. *Staphylococcus aureus*
E. *Streptococcus viridans*

28.2

Aisha, a 14-year-old girl, has developed a right-sided limp that has been present for 2 weeks. She is now complaining of pain in her right hip and knee. On examination, she has a temperature of 37.7°C. She is overweight (95th centile), with a body mass index of 26 kg/m². She has a decreased range of movement of the right hip. Blood tests, including a full-blood count and a C-reactive protein are taken and results are found to be normal.

Her hip X-ray is shown in Fig. 28.1 opposite.

What is the most likely diagnosis?

Select one answer only.

A. Osgood–Schlatter disease
B. Osteomyelitis

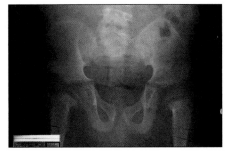

Figure 28.1

C. Perthes disease
D. Septic arthritis
E. Slipped capital femoral epiphysis

28.3

Zain is a 14-year-old boy who presents to the Emergency Department. He is a good footballer, and after training today he complained of pain in his left knee. He has had the pain for a while and it gets worse when he exercises. On examination there is swelling over the left tibial tuberosity. He is afebrile. There is no night pain or pain on waking.

What is the most likely diagnosis?

Select one answer only.

A. Osteomyelitis
B. Osgood–Schlatter disease
C. Perthes disease
D. Septic arthritis
E. Slipped capital femoral epiphysis

28.4

Edward, aged 3 years, woke up complaining of pain in his right leg. Yesterday he refused to play in the garden with his older brother, preferring to watch television. Since then he has become more unwell and his mother reports he is lethargic. On examination he has a temperature of 39°C, a heart rate of 180 beats/min, and a respiratory rate of 25 breaths/min. His right knee is red and swollen and he cries if it is extended or flexed. On further examination you note a small healing insect bite on his right ankle. He has no other medical problems and is not currently on any medication.

What is the most likely diagnosis?

Select one answer only.

A. Henoch–Schönlein purpura arthritis
B. Juvenile idiopathic arthritis
C. Osteomyelitis
D. Septic arthritis
E. Trauma

28.5
Karen, aged 5 years, presents to her general practitioner. She has been unwell for 2 weeks with lethargy, fever and painful wrists and knees. On examination she has a temperature of 38.5°C and a subtle erythematous rash on her trunk. You identify that several joints are swollen, warm, and painful to move, including the wrists, her right elbow, the knees, her left ankle and left hip. She has some cervical lymphadenopathy and her spleen is palpable. She has no previous medical problems and her mother has been giving her paracetamol. You perform some blood tests and get the following results:

- Hb (haemoglobin), 85 g/L; WBC (white blood count), 17×10^9/L; neutrophils, 10.4×10^9/L; platelets, 366×10^9/L
- blood film: normal, no atypical lymphocytes
- ESR (erythrocyte sedimentation rate): 70 mm/hour
- ANA (antinuclear antibody): negative
- double-stranded DNA: negative
- antistreptolysin O titre: normal.

What is the most likely diagnosis?

Select one answer only.

A. Acute lymphoblastic leukaemia
B. Epstein–Barr virus infection
C. Post-streptococcal arthritis
D. Systemic lupus erythematosus (SLE)
E. Systemic-onset juvenile idiopathic arthritis

28.6
William is an 8-year-old boy who presents with joint pain. His mother reports that since yesterday he has been refusing to walk, as his legs are so painful. On examination his temperature is 37°C and his heart rate is 100 beats/min. He is settled at rest and playing a computer game on his iPad. On further examination you notice a rash over his lower limbs, buttocks, and forearms (Fig. 28.2). The rash comprises some large (5–15 mm), red, raised lesions, and multiple pin-point lesions, which do not blanch on pressure. His peripheries are warm and he has a good pulse volume with a normal

capillary refill time. There is some generalized swelling around his knees and ankles. He has pain on passive movement of both knees and ankles.

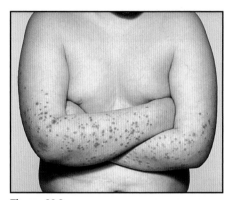

Figure 28.2

What is the most likely diagnosis?

Select one answer only.

A. Henoch–Schönlein purpura
B. Immune thrombocytopaenic purpura
C. Meningococcal septicaemia
D. Reactive arthritis (transient synovitis)
E. Systemic-onset juvenile idiopathic arthritis

28.7
Dominika is a 3-year-old girl. She presents with an acute onset limp which was not present on the previous day. Her mother reports that she was unwell 2 weeks ago with a coryzal illness. The pain is in her right leg and is present only on walking. On examination she has a temperature of 37°C. The hip and leg look normal but on passive movement of her right hip, there is decreased external rotation.

What is the most likely diagnosis from the list below?

Select one answer only.

A. Bone tumour
B. Perthes disease
C. Reactive arthritis (transient synovitis)
D. Septic arthritis
E. Slipped capital femoral epiphysis

28.8
You are asked to review Huw, a baby who is 24 hours old. He was born by vaginal delivery following a normal pregnancy. The midwife has noted that the baby's feet look abnormal. On examination the feet are turned inwards but appear to be of a normal size. On passive movement of the foot you are able to manipulate it so that it can be fully dorsiflexed to touch the front of the lower leg (neutral position).

What is the most likely diagnosis from the list given below?

Select one answer only.

A. Positional talipes equinovarus
B. Talipes calcaneovalgus
C. Talipes equinovarus
D. Tarsal coalition
E. Vertical talus

28.9

Harry is an 18-month-old boy. He is brought to the Emergency Department as he has stopped walking and his mother is worried his left leg is painful. On examination he will not weight bear, and cries when his left leg is moved passively. He is afebrile and the rest of his examination is normal, except that you think his sclera has a slight blue tinge. An X-ray is performed, which shows a fracture of his femur, but there is also a comment that the bones look osteoporotic. On further questioning from his mother, she cannot give any history of trauma or any incident that could have caused the fracture. On looking back through the notes you note that he broke his left arm 4 months ago and again his mother could not give any explanation as to why this had happened. Harry's older sister is with them and has her arm in a splint having recently fractured it.

What is the most likely diagnosis for Harry?

Select one answer only.

A. Accidental injury (unwitnessed)
B. Non-accidental injury
C. Osteogenesis imperfecta
D. Osteomyelitis
E. Osteopetrosis

28.10

John is an 8-year-old boy. He presents to the Emergency Department with a 5-day history of pain in his right leg. It has slowly been getting worse. He has not had a fever. There is no history of trauma. On examination he has a painful limp. He has a reduced range of movement of the right hip. He has no medical history of note, and has been taking ibuprofen for the pain, which has helped a little.

An X-ray of his pelvis is shown in Fig. 28.3.

Select the most likely diagnosis. Select one answer only.

A. Fractured femur
B. Osteosarcoma
C. Perthes disease
D. Reactive arthritis (transient synovitis)
E. Slipped capital femoral epiphysis

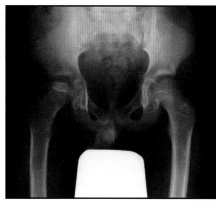

Figure 28.3

28.11

John is 14 years old. He presents to his general practitioner as he is conscious of his physical appearance. He is the tallest boy in his class and he does not like getting changed for sport at school because the other boys mock him. On examination his height is above the 98th centile, he has long fingers, and a wide arm span. You inspect his chest (Fig. 28.4).

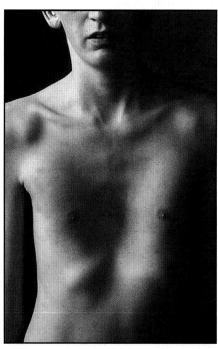

Figure 28.4

Select the most likely diagnosis.

A. Harrison's sulci
B. Kyphosis
C. Pectus excavatum
D. Pectus carinatum
E. Scoliosis

Questions: Extended Matching

28.12
For each of the following patients select the most likely diagnosis (A–K). Each option may be used once, more than once, or not at all.

A. Cellulitis
B. Fractured femur
C. Juvenile idiopathic arthritis
D. Osteomyelitis
E. Osteosarcoma
F. Perthes disease
G. Reactive arthritis (transient synovitis)
H. Septic arthritis
I. Slipped capital femoral epiphysis
J. Rheumatic fever
K. Vitamin D deficiency

28.12.1
Emma, aged 3½ years, presents to the Emergency Department. She has a 24-hour history of a limp and pain in her left thigh. There is no history of trauma. Her temperature is 38.9°C and her pulse is 150 beats/min. On examination the left thigh is swollen and held flexed and abducted. She holds it as still as possible and cries if it is moved. The upper leg is slightly red and is warmer to touch than the right leg. She has no other medical history and her mother has given some paracetamol, which had no effect on the pain.

28.12.2
The parents of Suliman, aged 18 months, bring him to their general practitioner. They are concerned because he has suddenly stopped walking. On examination he is miserable but apyrexial. His left thigh is swollen. There is no discoloration of the skin and it is not warm to touch. On inspection it appears that he is not moving his left foot, however, he withdraws it on tickling his foot, which leads him to cry. He is unable to weight bear. He has no other medical problem and is not on any medications.

28.12.3
Claire is 5 years old. She presents with a swollen joint. Her knee joint has been swollen for several days. There is some mild tenderness but she continues to walk, with a slight limp. Her mother reports that 3 weeks ago she had a bout of gastroenteritis associated with a fever. There were two episodes of bloody diarrhoea and she vomited once. Her symptoms resolved without

treatment. On examination she is afebrile. Her right knee is swollen with only mild tenderness on passive movements of the joint. There is no other medical history of note and she is not on any medication.

28.13
For each of the following patients with leg pain (A–L), select the most likely diagnosis. Each option may be used once, more than once, or not at all.

A. Acute lymphoblastic leukaemia
B. Chondromalacia patellae
C. Complex regional pain syndrome
D. Growing pains
E. Hypermobility
F. Osgood–Schlatter disease
G. Osteochondritis dissecans
H. Osteomyelitis
I. Scheuermann disease
J. Spondylolysis
K. Rickets
L. Tumour – osteoid osteoma

28.13.1
Milly, a 6-year-old girl, is taken to her general practitioner by her mother as she has started waking up at night and complaining that her legs hurt. This started about 2 months ago. She goes off to sleep okay but wakes up at around midnight and cries out. Her mother feels she is in pain and has to massage her legs before she will go back to sleep. On examination she looks well. Her legs look normal and she has a full range of movement around all the joints. The rest of her examination is normal.

28.13.2
Flora is a 12-year-old girl. She presents to the Emergency Department for the third time in 10 days. Her right ankle is extremely painful and she is unable to weight bear, and is brought into the department in a wheelchair. She was playing netball 10 days ago when the ball landed on her foot. Ever since then it has been painful and has been getting worse. She had an X-ray which showed no fracture. On examination she has extreme tenderness over the medial aspect of her foot, even when touched very lightly with a bit of cotton wool. The right foot feels slightly colder than the left foot, but her foot pulses are normal. She refuses to move the foot and will not let you try and move it for her as it is so painful. The rest of her examination is entirely normal and she is systemically well with no fever.

28.13.3
Suji, a 14-year-old girl, complains of pains in her knees when walking upstairs. She is otherwise well. She is free of pain whilst sitting in her chair, but complains of pain in both knees when asked to stand up. On examination you notice that she

has loss of the medial arch of her feet. She has no other medical problems and is not on any medication.

28.13.4
Joseph is a 14-year-old boy who presents to his general practitioner. He complains of pain and swelling in his right knee for several weeks. This is worse after playing football. On examination you note swelling over the tibial tuberosity. He has no other medical problems and has been taking paracetamol when the pain is present.

28.13.5
Craig is 5 years old and is complaining that his back hurts. This started about 4 weeks ago and his mother tried to ignore it as there was nothing to see and ibuprofen seemed to help. However, he has now started waking up at night crying out that his back is sore. He has not had a fever. His father suffers from back pain and is off work with it at the moment. On examination he is reluctant to move his back for you but there is no obvious tenderness over his spine and there is mild scoliosis. His neurological examination is normal.

28.14
For each of the following children, select the most likely diagnosis (A–J). Each option may be used once, more than once, or not at all.

A. Bow legs – normal variant
B. Bow legs – rickets
C. Developmental dysplasia of the hip – late diagnosis
D. Kyphosis
E. Normal variant of childhood
F. Pectus excavatum
G. Pectus carinatum
H. Perthes disease
I. Scoliosis
J. Slipped capital femoral epiphysis

28.14.1
Jack is a 14-month-old boy. He has only recently started walking. His mother brings him to his general practitioner as she is concerned that he walks with a limp. You examine his gait and he has a painless limp of his right leg. He has asymmetry of the skin folds around his right thigh and his right hip cannot be fully abducted. He has no other medical history. He was born by elective caesarean section because of breech presentation.

28.14.2
Zahra is a 4-year-old Asian girl. Her mother is concerned about her leg shape. On examination you notice that on standing, the knees are very widely spaced with the feet held together. On completing the musculoskeletal examination, you notice that she has swollen wrist joints. There is no other medical history of note and she is not on any medications.

28.14.3
Rachel, a 2-year-old girl, is seen for a developmental check by the health visitor. She is walking on her own but the health visitor notes that she has flat feet while she is walking. She tries to get Rachel to stand on her tiptoes but she cannot. When she passively extends her big toe an arch is demonstrated.

28.14.4
Alliah is a 2½-year-old girl. She is seen in the paediatric outpatient department because her mother is worried about her walking, as she usually walks on tiptoes. She was born by normal vaginal delivery at 37 weeks. She started to walk at 15 months. She never crawled but did bottom shuffle. On examination of her gait she mostly walks and runs on tiptoes, and her mother confirms she has done this ever since she started walking. However, she can walk on her heels if asked to do so. General examination of her legs demonstrates normal tone and reflexes.

Answers: Single Best Answer

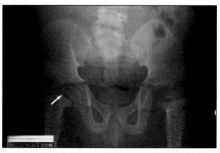

Figure 28.5

28.1

A. *Haemophilus influenza*
Haemophilus influenzae may cause osteomyelitis, particularly in unimmunized children but is an uncommon causative organism.

B. *Mycobacterium tuberculosis*
Tuberculosis may cause osteomyelitis but is an uncommon cause in the UK and presents more insidiously. It might be difficult to exclude. Consider a chest X-ray and Mantoux test or IGRA (interferon-gamma release assay) if his condition does not resolve.

C. *Salmonella typhi*
In sickle cell anaemia, there is an increased risk of *Salmonella* osteomyelitis.

D. *Staphylococcus aureus* ⊘
Correct. Amir is most likely to have osteomyelitis, usually caused by *Staphylococcus aureus*, but other pathogens include *Streptococcus*. In sickle cell anaemia, there is an increased risk of *Staphylococcus* and *Salmonella* osteomyelitis.

E. *Streptococcus viridans*
Most infections are caused by *Staphylococcus aureus* but other pathogens include group A *Streptococcus* species.

28.2

A. Osgood–Schlatter disease
Osgood–Schlatter disease affects the knees.

B. Osteomyelitis
Osteomyelitis is less likely as she is not systemically unwell, for example there is no fever.

C. Perthes disease
Perthes disease usually affects children aged 5–10 years. There is degeneration of the femoral head – which is not seen here.

D. Septic arthritis
Septic arthritis is less likely as she is not systemically unwell.

E. Slipped capital femoral epiphysis ⊘
Correct. She has a slipped capital femoral epiphysis (also known as slipped upper femoral epiphysis). This results in displacement of the epiphysis of the femoral head postero-inferiorly (Fig. 28.5, arrow). It is most common at 10–15 years of age during the adolescent growth spurt, particularly in obese individuals.

28.3

A. Osteomyelitis
Would be a very unusual cause, particularly without fever.

B. Osgood–Schlatter disease ⊘
Correct. This is osteochondritis of the patellar tendon insertion at the knee, often affecting adolescent males who are physically active (particularly football or basketball). It usually presents with knee pain after exercise, localized tenderness and sometimes swelling over the tibial tuberosity. There is often hamstring tightness. It is bilateral in 25–50% of cases.

C. Perthes disease
Whilst pain might be referred to the knees from the hips, it is unlikely in this boy.

D. Septic arthritis
Fever absent – and he can still weight bear.

E. Slipped capital femoral epiphysis
Affects the hip. There would not be swelling over the tibial tuberosity.

28.4

A. Henoch–Schönlein purpura arthritis
The arthritis of Henoch–Schönlein purpura would usually be accompanied by a rash and a high fever would not be present.

B. Juvenile idiopathic arthritis
Does not usually present so acutely with a single red swollen joint.

C. Osteomyelitis
The main differential diagnosis.

D. Septic arthritis ⊘
Correct. Septic arthritis. Needs to be differentiated from osteomyelitis. Edward's knee joint itself is red and swollen, with pain on movement, making septic arthritis more likely. An ultrasound and aspiration of the joint should be performed to confirm this.

E. Trauma
There is no history of trauma.

28.5

A. Acute lymphoblastic leukaemia
Acute lymphoblastic leukaemia needs to be considered, but is less likely as Karen has numerous joints affected and the blood film is normal.

B. Epstein–Barr virus infection
Epstein–Barr virus is unlikely as it rarely causes widespread arthritis.

C. Post-streptococcal arthritis
Post-streptococcal arthritis is unlikely as the antistreptolysin O titre is normal, although a repeat blood test is required to confirm that the titre remains low.

D. Systemic lupus erythematosus (SLE)
SLE may have similar clinical features but is unlikely as the ANA (antinuclear antibody) and double-stranded DNA are negative. SLE is also very uncommon at this age.

E. Systemic-onset juvenile idiopathic arthritis ⊘
Correct. Systemic-onset juvenile idiopathic arthritis is the most likely diagnosis, as she has a systemic illness, polyarthritis (more than four joints) and a salmon-pink rash. The raised neutrophil count and markedly raised ESR are consistent with the diagnosis.

28.6
A. Henoch–Schönlein purpura ⊘
Correct. Henoch–Schönlein purpura is the most common vasculitis of childhood, and presents with a purpuric rash over the lower legs and buttocks, but which can also involve the extensor surface of the elbows. It is often associated with arthritis of the ankles or knees. In this case the child presented with the arthritis rather than the rash. Other features are abdominal pain, haematuria and proteinuria.

B. Immune thrombocytopaenic purpura
The raised rash suggests a vasculitis rather than just low platelets. Also the distribution in Henoch–Schönlein purpura and immune thrombocytopaenic purpura is different.

C. Meningococcal septicaemia
Meningococcal sepsis is unlikely as he is afebrile, and the purpura is restricted to his lower limbs and elbows.

D. Reactive arthritis (transient synovitis)
Reactive arthritis is unlikely as there is usually a preceding or accompanying infection, and the rash would not have this distribution and certainly would not be purpuric.

E. Systemic-onset juvenile idiopathic arthritis
Systemic-onset juvenile idiopathic arthritis is accompanied by a high fever in a child who is systemically unwell; the salmon-pink coloured rash is widespread and blanches.

28.7
A. Bone tumour
A bone tumour is rare at this age and usually presents insidiously.

B. Perthes disease
Perthes disease usually occurs in older children.

C. Reactive arthritis (transient synovitis) ⊘
Correct. This is the most common cause of acute hip pain in children. It occurs in children aged

2–12 years of age. It often follows or is accompanied by a viral infection.
Presentation is with sudden onset of pain in the hip or a limp. There is no pain at rest, but there is decreased range of movement, particularly external rotation.

D. Septic arthritis
Septic arthritis of the hip joint can be difficult to differentiate from reactive arthritis (transient synovitis) but is far less common. Children with septic arthritis are usually systemically unwell and have a fever. There may be erythema and swelling around the joint, but this may not be evident at the hip. There is severe pain on any movement of the leg, and refusal to weight bear. If necessary, a normal ultrasound scan and C-reactive protein evaluation will help exclude it.

E. Slipped capital femoral epiphysis
Slipped capital femoral epiphysis usually occurs in older children.

28.8
A. Positional talipes equinovarus ⊘
Correct. This is a common problem and is caused by intrauterine compression. The foot is of normal size, the deformity is mild and can be corrected to the neutral position with passive manipulation.

B. Talipes calcaneovalgus
Talipes calcaneovalgus is a fixed bony deformity, in which the foot is everted and dorsiflexed.

C. Talipes equinovarus
Talipes equinovarus is a fixed bony deformity, in which the foot is inverted and supinated. Passive movement to a normal, neutral position is not possible. See Figs. 28.5 and 28.6 in Illustrated Textbook of Paediatrics for more details.

D. Tarsal coalition
Tarsal coalition is a diagnosis made in adolescent years.

E. Vertical talus
Vertical talus is in children with rocker bottom feet who often have other congenital abnormalities.

28.9
A. Accidental injury (unwitnessed)
Possible, but why the recurrent pattern?

B. Non-accidental injury
Although non-accidental injury needs to be considered, the abnormality of the bones on X-ray makes osteogenesis imperfecta more likely. In clinical settings child protection concerns must be addressed in parallel with investigation for osteogenesis imperfecta and other medical conditions.

C. Osteogenesis imperfecta ⊘
Correct. Harry is likely to have osteogenesis imperfecta (type 1). It presents with fractures in early childhood and the bones look osteoporotic

on X-ray. The children often have blue sclera but this can be difficult to identify with confidence. The condition is autosomal dominant and it is likely his older sister Amy has it as well.

D. Osteomyelitis
Osteomyelitis does present with a painful leg, but would usually be associated with fever and redness over the area. The X-ray is usually normal at presentation.

E. Osteopetrosis
Osteopetrosis is also an autosomal dominant disease that can present in its milder form with fractures, but the bones look dense on X-ray.

28.10
A. Fractured femur
Always a possibility, but the X-ray is showing a specific change in the femoral head.

B. Osteosarcoma
Worth considering but the destruction here is of the femoral head.

C. Perthes disease ⊘
Correct. John has Perthes disease. This affects boys five times more frequently than girls. It usually presents between the age of 5 and 10 years. The X-ray Fig. 28.6 confirms the diagnosis with flattening of the right femoral capital epiphysis. When in doubt about the X-ray, compare both hips.

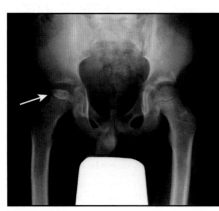

Figure 28.6

D. Reactive arthritis (transient synovitis)
The X-ray would be normal.

E. Slipped capital femoral epiphysis
More common in overweight teenage girls.

28.11
A. Harrison's sulci
This would lead to indentation at points of insertion of the diaphragm.

B. Kyphosis
The spine is 'bent over'.

C. Pectus excavatum ⊘
Correct. Pectus excavatum is also known as 'hollow chest' or 'funnel chest'. This boy probably has Marfan syndrome, but it also occurs in otherwise normal children.

D. Pectus carinatum
This is also known as a 'pigeon chest' and results in a protrusion of the sternum.

E. Scoliosis
There is lateral curvature of the spine and rib humping when bending over.

Answers: Extended Matching

Answer 28.12.1
H. Septic arthritis
It can be difficult to clinically differentiate between osteomyelitis and septic arthritis. In this child, the very acute history and flexed and abducted position of the thigh at rest suggest septic arthritis. Ultrasound (and diagnostic aspiration), blood tests for culture and tests for inflammatory markers should be performed and intravenous antibiotics started. It is important to not delay treatment as this can lead to permanent damage to the joint and urgent orthopaedic review should be sought.

Answer 28.12.2
B. Fractured femur
A fractured femur may be accidental but non-accidental injury needs to be considered in all unexplained fractures. In osteomyelitis and septic arthritis he would be unwell with a fever, the left thigh would be warm and discoloured, and he would be unwilling to move the limb at all.

Answer 28.12.3
G. Reactive arthritis (transient synovitis)
She has a reactive arthritis. As this followed an episode of gastroenteritis with bloody diarrhoea, it is likely to be due to enteric bacteria (e.g. *Campylobacter*).

Answer 28.13.1
D. Growing pains
This condition is poorly understood, but the child has episodes of generalized pain in the lower limbs, which often wakes them from sleep. It occurs in preschool-age and school-age children. The pain is symmetrical in the lower limbs. The pain is not present at the start of the day, and physical activity is not limited. The physical examination is entirely normal. Hypermobility can cause pain in the limbs but this child did not demonstrate any hypermobility of the joints.

Answer 28.13.2
C. Complex regional pain syndrome
Flora is likely to have a localized complex regional pain syndrome, which often presents in a single foot or ankle after minor trauma. In addition to severe pain, there may be hyperaesthesia (increased sensitivity to stimuli), allodynia (pain from a stimulus that does not normally produce pain) and the affected part (often a foot or hand) may be cool to touch with swelling and mottling.

Answer 28.13.3
B. *Chondromalacia patellae*
There is softening of the articular cartilage of the patella. It most often affects adolescent females, causing pain when the patella is tightly apposed to the femoral condyles, as in standing up from sitting or on walking up stairs. It is often associated with hypermobility and flat feet, suggesting a biomechanical component to the aetiology.

Answer 28.13.4
F. Osgood–Schlatter disease
This is an osteochondritis of the patellar tendon insertion at the knee, often affecting adolescent males who are physically active (particularly football or basketball). It usually presents with knee pain after exercise, localized tenderness, and sometimes swelling over the tibial tuberosity. It is bilateral in 25–50% of cases.

Answer 28.13.5
L. Tumour – osteoid osteoma
Craig may have a benign tumour, an osteoid osteoma. It presents with back pain, which is worse at night. Back pain in young children must be taken seriously, as it is uncommon. Red flag features include a young age, waking at night, fever, weight loss and focal neurological signs. Osteomyelitis of the back can occur and would present with pain but is usually associated with a fever, systemic upset and tenderness over the area.

Answer 28.14.1
C. Developmental dysplasia of the hip – late diagnosis
Jack has developmental dysplasia of the hip. This is usually identified on one of the two hip screening checks (birth and 6–8 weeks) babies receive in the UK. He was at increased risk as he was a breech presentation. Occasionally, it is not identified, as examination is not 100% sensitive. Late presentation is with a painless limp.

Answer 28.14.2
B. Bow legs – rickets
This girl has bow legs (genu varum), which would be a common variant of normal up until 3 years of age. The finding of swollen wrists leads to the diagnosis of rickets. This girl should have blood tests to confirm the diagnosis and be started on vitamin D supplementation along with dietary advice and advice regarding increasing sunlight exposure.

Answer 28.14.3
E. Normal variant of childhood
This is a normal variant of childhood. Toddlers learning to walk usually have flat feet due to flatness of the medial longitudinal arch and the presence of a fat pad, which disappears as the child gets older. An arch can usually be demonstrated on standing on tiptoe, or by passively extending the big toe. Marked flat feet are common in hypermobility. A fixed flat foot, often painful, may indicate a congenital tarsal coalition and requires an orthopaedic opinion. Rachel is unable to stand on her tiptoes, not because of a pathological condition but because children are unable to do so at this age.

Answer 28.14.4
E. Normal variant of childhood
Toe walking is common in young children and may become persistent, usually from habit. The child can walk normally on request. Children with mild cerebral palsy can present with toe walking but an increase in tone would be found on examination. In older boys, Duchenne muscular dystrophy should be excluded.

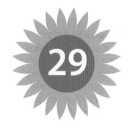

Neurological disorders

Questions: Single Best Answer

29.1

Annette is a 15-year-old girl who complains of worsening daily occipital headaches. They occur mainly in the mornings and sometimes wake her from sleep. Her mother says she is doing less well at school than previously and has become a difficult and grumpy teenager. She sometimes vomits in the mornings. She has no other medical problems though she is on the oral contraceptive pill.

What is the most likely diagnosis?

Select one answer only.

A. Idiopathic intracranial hypertension
B. Migraine
C. Medication side-effect
D. Tension headache
E. Raised intracranial pressure due to a space-occupying lesion

29.2

Gerald is a 10-year-old boy. He is seen in the special school clinic with his mother, who is just recovering from cataract surgery. He has moderate learning difficulties and is teased because of his marked facial weakness. He is unable to walk long distances. His mother says that he struggles to release things once he grabs them. He has no other medical problems. He has not had any investigations performed.

Select the most useful diagnostic test from the list.

Select one answer only.

A. DNA testing for trinucleotide repeat expansion
B. Electromyography (EMG)
C. Muscle biopsy
D. Nerve conduction studies
E. Serum creatine kinase

29.3

Olive is a 5-year-old girl who had a myelomeningocele repaired shortly after birth. She uses a wheelchair for mobility. She has a 4-day history of fever, lethargy, vomiting and abdominal pain. She normally opens her bowels twice a week and does intermittent urinary catheterization three times a day with the help of her mother but despite this she is dribbling urine.

What is the most likely cause of her new symptoms.

Select one answer only.

A. Constipation
B. Hydrocephalus
C. Hypertension and renal failure
D. Tethering of the spinal cord
E. Urinary tract infection

29.4

Angelo, a 15-month-old boy, had been unwell with a runny nose and cough for a day when his father brings him to the Emergency Department. At lunch he suddenly became stiff, his eyes rolled upwards and both his arms and legs started jerking for 2 minutes. He felt very hot at the time. When examined 2 hours later, he has recovered fully. This is the first time this has happened. He has a normal neurological examination and is acquiring his developmental milestones normally. He has no other medical problems. The triage nurse performed a blood glucose test, which indicated a glucose level of 4.2 mmol/L (within normal range).

What would be the most appropriate investigation?

A. CT scan of the brain
B. ECG
C. EEG (electroencephalography)
D. No investigation required
E. Oral glucose tolerance test

29.5

Pamela is an 8-year-old girl with recurrent seizures. She has three or four seizures a month, where she lets out a cry, her arms and legs become stiff, her eyes roll upwards and then she jerks her arms and legs. This lasts about 3 minutes. Afterwards she sleeps for 2 hours and is then back to normal. She is doing well at school but is sometimes missing school because of her seizures. She is currently not on any medication and has no other medical problems.

What would be the best intervention for this child?

Select one answer only.

A. Anti-epileptic drug therapy
B. Home schooling
C. Ketogenic diet
D. No intervention required
E. Vagal nerve stimulation

29.6
Alan is a 7-month-old male infant who was preterm, born at 28 weeks' gestation, birthweight 970 g, and whose family recently arrived in this country. He is seen in a paediatric clinic because of vomiting. He had been seen regularly by a doctor who was treating him for gastro-oesophageal reflux. He has always vomited but this has been getting worse and his mother has noticed his eye movements are not normal. His examination findings can be seen in Fig. 29.1.

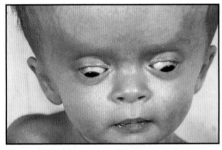

Figure 29.1 (Courtesy of Dr Tony Hulse).

What is the most likely underlying cause for these findings?

Select one answer only.

A. Aqueduct stenosis
B. Intraventricular haemorrhage
C. Meningitis
D. Posterior fossa neoplasm
E. Subarachnoid haemorrhage

29.7
Sharon is an 11-year-old girl who has had occasional headaches for the last 3 months. Today was her first day at secondary school. During maths class she developed her usual throbbing left-sided headache, associated with nausea. Over the next hour, she lost her temporal vision in her right eye and found she only had minimal movement in her right arm. The left side of her mouth was drooping. Her parents were called, who rushed her to hospital. She is now feeling much better, has normal vision and can move her arm, although she has some residual weakness of her mouth. She has no significant medical history except some episodes of abdominal pain as a younger child. Her mother tells you that she also suffers from headaches.

What is the most likely diagnosis?

Select one answer only.

A. Idiopathic intracranial hypertension
B. Migraine
C. Raised intracranial pressure due to a space-occupying lesion
D. Subarachnoid haemorrhage
E. Tension headache

29.8
Aparna is a 2-year-old girl of Indian ethnicity who lives in the UK. She presents to her general practitioner as she has been unsteady on her feet for a day, having had diarrhoea during the previous week. On examination she is afebrile, has reduced muscle power and tone and no tendon reflexes can be elicited in her lower limbs. She is referred urgently to the paediatric hospital and 6 hours later she is unable to stand and the tendon reflexes in her upper limbs are now absent. She has no other medical problems and has been fully immunized.

What is the most likely diagnosis?

Select one answer only.

A. Guillain–Barré syndrome
B. Myasthenia gravis
C. Myotonic dystrophy
D. Poliomyelitis
E. Spinal muscular atrophy

29.9
Jordain is a 7-year-old child born in Yemen who presents to the children's outpatient department. His mother is concerned regarding a number of skin marks, which she has noticed over the last year. She was not initially concerned about them, but they are becoming more numerous and larger in size. She reports that Jordain's father also had similar skin marks before he passed away from 'cancer'. On examining Jordain you see the skin lesions shown in Fig. 29.2. He also has a large number of freckles in his axilla region. He has no other medical problems and is not on any medications.

What is the most likely diagnosis?

Select one answer only.

A. Ataxia telangiectasia
B. Friedreich ataxia
C. Neurofibromatosis
D. Sturge–Weber syndrome
E. Tuberous sclerosis

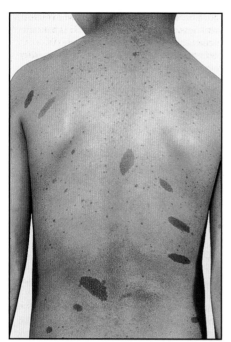

Figure 29.2 (Courtesy of Dr Graham Clayden).

29.10

Gregor is born at term. It was a normal pregnancy though the mother did not have any antenatal ultrasound examinations as she was against medical procedures. He was born by vaginal delivery. Immediately, the midwife noticed the lesion shown in Fig. 29.3.

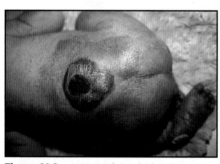

Figure 29.3

Which of the supplements listed would have reduced the risk of this problem if taken by the mother periconceptually?

Select one answer only.

A. Folic acid
B. Iron
C. Vitamin A
D. Vitamin B$_{12}$
E. Vitamin D

29.11

Antonia, a 5-year-old girl, is seen by her general practitioner. Her mother and school teacher have noticed she has episodes where she stops her activity for a few seconds, stares blankly ahead and then resumes the activity as if she had never stopped. These episodes happen many times a day. She has no other medical problems and there is no family history of note. The EEG during an episode is shown in Fig. 29.4.

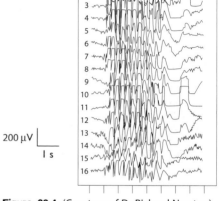

200 µV

1 s

Figure 29.4 (Courtesy of Dr Richard Newton).

Choose the most likely diagnosis.

Select one answer only.

A. Childhood Rolandic epilepsy (benign epilepsy with centro-temporal spikes)
B. Childhood absence epilepsy
C. Juvenile myoclonic epilepsy
D. Lennox-Gastaut syndrome
E. Infantile spasms (West syndrome)

29.12

Vijay is a 5-month-old infant who has been seen repeatedly by his general practitioner because of colic. His mother brings him to the Accident and Emergency department as he is having episodes of suddenly throwing his head and arms forward. These episodes occur in repetitive bursts. His mother thinks they may be something more than just colic, as he is now not smiling or supporting his head as well as he did previously. He was born at term by normal vaginal delivery and has no other medical problems. His EEG is shown in Fig. 29.5.

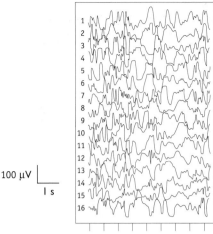

100 μV

1 s

Figure 29.5 (Courtesy of Dr Richard Newton).

Choose the most likely diagnosis.

Select one answer only.

A. Juvenile myoclonic epilepsy
B. Lennox-Gastaut syndrome
C. Childhood Rolandic epilepsy (benign epilepsy with centro-temporal spikes)
D. Childhood absence epilepsy
E. Infantile spasms (West syndrome)

Questions: Extended Matching

29.13

For each of the scenarios (A–N) of children who have had a funny turn, pick the most likely diagnosis from the list. Each answer can be used once, more than once, or not at all.

A. Benign paroxysmal vertigo
B. Blue breath-holding spells (expiratory apnoea syncope)
C. Cardiac arrhythmia
D. Childhood absence epilepsy
E. Hypoglycaemia
F. Intracranial haemorrhage
G. Migraine
H. Narcolepsy
I. Night terrors
J. Non-epileptic attack disorder (pseudoseizure)
K. Reflex asystolic syncope (reflex anoxic seizure)
L. Syncope
M. Tic disorder
N. Tonic–clonic seizure

29.13.1

Emily, a normally fit and healthy 3-year-old girl, is rushed to the Emergency Department. She had been playing at nursery and had banged her head against a door. Almost immediately she went very pale and stiff and had jerking movements of her arms and legs for 20 seconds. Afterwards she was groggy for a few minutes, but is now back to her usual self. This has not happened before. Her mother is very distressed and now reports feeling faint herself. The triage nurse has performed a blood glucose which indicates a glucose level of 4.1 mmol/L (within normal range).

29.13.2

Jennifer, an 11-year-old girl, is brought to the Emergency Department after collapsing at school. Her teacher described her standing in assembly, becoming pale and collapsing to the floor. She had a couple of jerking movements of her limbs lasting a few seconds. She returned to normal promptly. Jennifer says that she had not eaten breakfast that morning, and experienced a sensation of feeling hot, a black curtain coming in front of her eyes, sounds becoming distant and feeling dizzy. The school nurse did a blood glucose, which indicated a glucose level of 3.5 mmol/L (within the normal range). She has had two episodes similar to this in the past but has not presented to hospital before. She has no other medical problems.

29.13.3

Bosco is an active 7-year-old black Caribbean boy, who was referred to the outpatient department with a history of collapse. He collapses during football practice or when he is playing outside with his siblings. This has happened at least six times in the last 3 months. His mother says that he suddenly becomes pale, loses consciousness and then slowly comes around. He has no medical history of note and has never had any investigations. His father died suddenly at the age of 34 years.

29.13.4

Rene is a lively 2-year-old boy who is seen in the acute paediatric assessment unit, having had an episode of turning blue and collapsing. This is not the first time that this has happened. He recovers quickly after these events. During the consultation his mother repeatedly gives him sweets to keep him calm. These episodes only occur when he is crying and this has led to his mother trying to avoid anything that will upset him. He has no other medical problems. His blood glucose today is 4.9 mmol/L.

29.13.5

Dora is an 8-year-old girl who attends the outpatient department. Her mother is worried because she used to be top of the class, but is not doing as well at school this year. Whilst in clinic, you notice that Dora has an episode where she suddenly stops what she is doing, stares ahead whilst flickering her eyelids for a couple of seconds and then resumes her previous activity as if nothing had happened. You ask her to blow out an imaginary candle, and the same thing happens again. She is growing normally and is otherwise fit and well.

29.14
For each scenario below (A–H), choose the most likely diagnosis. Each diagnosis can be used once, more than once, or not at all.

A. Childhood Rolandic epilepsy (benign epilepsy with centro-temporal spikes)
B. Childhood absence epilepsy
C. Juvenile myoclonic epilepsy
D. Lennox–Gastaut syndrome
E. Infantile spasms (West syndrome)

29.14.1
Damasco is a 6-year-old black boy who presents in the paediatric clinic. He has been referred because his brother, with whom he shares a room, has woken his parents early in the morning on several occasions complaining that Damasco is making unusual sounds and drooling from his mouth. By the time his parents come to the room Damasco is jerking his upper and lower limbs rhythmically. This lasts for 1–2 minutes. Afterwards Damasco complains of a funny sensation on the left side of his mouth, and then goes back to sleep. He is doing well at school and clinical examination is normal. He has no other medical problems.

29.14.2
Jude is a 14-year-old boy who is on treatment for generalised tonic–clonic and absence seizures. He attends a routine clinic appointment complaining of regularly spilling his tea in the morning because his arm jerks involuntarily. These jerks are worse if he has stayed up late the night before. He is doing relatively well at school.

29.14.3
Andrew is a 5-year-old boy with severe learning difficulties who attends a special school. He is seen in his review clinic. His epilepsy is difficult to control and he is on two different antiepileptic drugs. He has several different types of seizures: sudden stiffening of his limbs causing him to fall, episodes of staring blankly ahead for up to 30 seconds before resuming previous activities, and episodes of his head dropping with a brief loss of consciousness. He is fed via a gastrostomy and has chronic drooling.

29.15
In the following clinical histories (A–I) choose the sign that is being described. Each finding can be used once, more than once, or not at all.

A. Babinski's sign
B. Brudzinski's sign
C. Chorea
D. Clonus
E. Dyskinesia
F. Fogs' sign
G. Gower's sign
H. Kernig's sign
I. Romberg's sign

29.15.1
Ahmed is a 5-year-old boy who presents to the outpatient clinic with weakness. His parents report that he finds it difficult to climb the stairs at home. This has been becoming progressively worse over the preceding 6–12 months. He is playing on the carpet with his brother when his mother calls him over. He has to roll from his back onto his front in order to stand up.

29.15.2
Christopher attends outpatient clinic for his routine follow-up. He is a 3-year-old boy who did not breathe at birth. Following resuscitation, he required intensive care for the first 5 days of life. He now has increased tone and reflexes in his right upper and lower limbs. On rubbing a blunt instrument up the lateral side of his right foot there is extension of the greater toe and fanning of his toes.

29.15.3
Sayeed is an 8-year-old Pakistani boy who has developed muscle weakness. His mother reports that he has poor coordination at home and at school. His speech has also recently become slurred. His problems have come on slowly over the last 12–18 months. He has no other medical history and is not taking any medications. On examination you notice that he has wasting of his calves.

When standing upright with his legs together and closing his eyes he becomes unsteady and starts to sway.

29.15.4
Jane is an 11-year-old girl who presents to the outpatient department. She complains that she finds it difficult to play sports such as basketball. In particular, she finds it difficult to run and coordinate her arm movements. She was born at 32 weeks' gestation and discharged from the neonatal service at 2 years of age as her development was normal. Her neurological examination appears to be normal except when you are examining her gait. On heel walking her left arm moves into a flexed position.

29.15.5
Paolo is a 7-year-old boy who presents to the Accident and Emergency department with fever. His mother reports that this has been present for the last 8 hours and that he is sleepy and wants to sleep in a dark room. He has no other medical history. On examination you note that he is photophobic. Whilst he is lying on the couch you flex his right knee and hip to 90°. On fully extending the knee, he complains of pain and arches on his back.

Answers: Single Best Answer

29.1

A. Idiopathic intracranial hypertension
Idiopathic intracranial hypertension also presents with features of raised intracranial pressure but is less likely to affect her behaviour and school performance, though they can be difficult to differentiate on clinical history alone.

B. Migraine
Migraine leads to asymmetrical features and typically the headaches are relieved by sleep.

C. Medication side-effect
Analgesia overuse can cause daily headache and is a common cause of chronic daily headache but this is not reported. This must always be included in the history. Sometimes parents are unaware that paracetamol is being taken frequently.

D. Tension headache
Although these headaches are very common, they are often at the end of the day. Rarely do they wake one from sleep.

E. Raised intracranial pressure due to a space-occupying lesion ⊘
Correct. This girl has raised intracranial pressure due to a space-occupying lesion. The headaches are worsening, and occur when lying down and wake her from sleep. Raised intracranial pressure is associated with morning vomiting. There is also behaviour change and worsening educational performance. The VI (abducens) cranial nerve has a long intracranial course and is often affected when there is raised pressure, resulting in a squint with diplopia and inability to abduct the eye beyond the midline. It is a false localising sign. Other nerves are affected depending on the site of lesion.

29.2

A. DNA testing for trinucleotide repeat expansion ⊘
Correct. The most useful diagnostic test here would be DNA testing for trinucleotide repeat expansion of myotonic dystrophy. The clinical history suggests myotonic dystrophy because of his learning difficulties, myotonia, facial weakness and limb weakness. It was dominantly inherited from his mother, who has cataracts as a result.

B. Electromyography (EMG)
You can test for the myotonia clinically rather than using electromyography, so DNA testing is the test most likely to give you the diagnosis.

C. Muscle biopsy
Muscle biopsies are performed when one needs to differentiate between muscle and neuronal pathology.

D. Nerve conduction studies
Difficult, costly and painful.

E. Serum creatine kinase
Serum creatine kinase is helpful in diagnosing muscular dystrophies, such as Duchenne.

29.3

A. Constipation
The constipation is not a new symptom but does predispose Olive to urinary tract infection.

B. Hydrocephalus
Hydrocephalus would cause lethargy and vomiting, but not the other symptoms.

C. Hypertension and renal failure
This is insidious and often presents as an incidental finding or with faltering growth.

D. Tethering of the spinal cord
Would not cause fever.

E. Urinary tract infection ⊘
Correct. Olive had a myelomeningocele that has caused a neurogenic bladder (she has to use catheterization to maintain continence) and neurogenic bowel dysfunction (she is usually constipated). A neurogenic bladder predisposes to developing a urinary tract infection, due to the stagnant urine lying in the bladder. Her symptoms of fever, abdominal pain, vomiting, and urinary incontinence are most likely to be due to a urinary tract infection.

29.4

A. CT scan of the brain
Persistent signs, particularly asymmetric ones, should prompt imaging.

B. ECG
Why the fever? Cardiac causes usually occur 'out of the blue' or following a specific trigger: exercise (hypertrophic obstructive cardiomyopathy) or shock (ventricular tachycardia).

C. EEG (electroencephalography)
Will be 'abnormal' in a significant proportion of normal children. This will lead to significant 'overdiagnosis' of epilepsy. Not indicated here.

D. No investigation required ⊘
Correct. Angelo had a simple febrile seizure, secondary to a respiratory tract infection. A febrile seizure is a clinical diagnosis and does not require investigation. Indeed, there is no confirmatory test.

E. Oral glucose tolerance test
This is not required as the blood glucose is normal. It is rarely required in children to diagnose diabetes.

29.5

A. Anti-epileptic drug therapy ⊘
Correct. This child should be started on an anti-epileptic drug. Pamela has recurrent generalised tonic–clonic seizures which are affecting her quality of life as she is missing school.

B. Home schooling
The solution to her missing school is control of her seizures.

C. Ketogenic diet
Ketogenic diets are sometimes used in children with intractable seizures.

D. No intervention required
The seizures are impacting upon schooling and quality of life.

E. Vagal nerve stimulation
Vagal nerve stimulation is used in certain children with intractable seizures.

29.6

A. Aqueduct stenosis
Possible but in view of prematurity another diagnosis is more likely.

B. Intraventricular haemorrhage ⊘
Correct. This child has hydrocephalus, and the most likely underlying cause is intraventricular haemorrhage from his prematurity. This results in impairment of drainage and reabsorption of CSF leading to post-haemorrhagic hydrocephalus. The figure shows his large head and sun-setting eyes, which, together with the vomiting, are all clinical features of hydrocephalus. He will also have an increasing head circumference, which will cross centile lines.

C. Meningitis
There is no fever or clinical features of sepsis or meningitis, which makes an infection unlikely.

D. Posterior fossa neoplasm
The eyes show features of sun-setting, not a cranial nerve palsy or squint characteristic of posterior fossa neoplasms. The history is suggestive of post-haemorrhagic hydrocephalus.

E. Subarachnoid haemorrhage
Not typical in preterm infants.

29.7

A. Idiopathic intracranial hypertension
Idiopathic intracranial hypertension would typically be worse on lying and/or straining. Often there is papilloedema.

B. Migraine ⊘
Correct. The headache is typical of a migraine, being unilateral and throbbing, and associated with nausea. However, this is a complicated migraine because it is associated with neurological phenomena (monoplegia and hemianopia) and

this necessitates neuroimaging to exclude a vascular abnormality or structural problem.

C. Raised intracranial pressure due to a space-occupying lesion
No red flags.

D. Subarachnoid haemorrhage
A subarachnoid haemorrhage is rare in a child of this age. Besides, the pain is often occipital and the neurological symptoms would not improve over this period.

E. Tension headache
A tension headache would be symmetrical, and the pain is not typically throbbing. In tension headaches there would not be weakness or visual disturbance.

29.8

A. Guillain–Barré syndrome ⊘
Correct. Guillain–Barré syndrome (post-infectious polyneuropathy). The classical presentation is with ascending weakness. It may follow campylobacter gastroenteritis. She must be closely monitored, as a serious complication is respiratory failure. To monitor her respiratory function, you can ask her to cough (or sing) to assess diaphragmatic function and involvement of the nerves supplying the chest muscles.

B. Myasthenia gravis
Myasthenia gravis presents as abnormal muscle fatigability, which improves with rest or anticholinesterase drugs. It is incredibly rare!

C. Myotonic dystrophy
Aparna's illness is an acute neuropathy.

D. Poliomyelitis
Poliomyelitis is a very important differential diagnosis here, but as the child is immunized and as polio has been eradicated in the UK it becomes far less likely. It is on the verge of eradication globally.

E. Spinal muscular atrophy
Spinal muscular atrophy is an autosomal recessive group of disorders causing degeneration of the anterior horn cells, leading to progressive weakness and wasting of skeletal muscles. They are chronic disorders and would not present acutely as in this child.

29.9

A. Ataxia telangiectasia
The skin lesions in ataxia telangiectasia are small dilated blood vessels near the surface of the skin or the mucous membranes.

B. Friedreich ataxia
Friedreich ataxia does not present with skin lesions.

C. Neurofibromatosis ⊘
Correct. The lesions seen in the image are café-au-lait spots. This is an autosomal dominant

disorder. There are criteria for making the diagnosis. This boy meets the diagnosis as he has six or more café-au-lait spots, has axilla freckles and it is likely he has a family history, related to his father.

D. Sturge–Weber syndrome
In Sturge–Weber syndrome there is a port-wine stain present on the face.

E. Tuberous sclerosis
In tuberous sclerosis there are a number of different skin lesions: depigmented, 'ash leaf'-shaped patches, which fluoresce under ultraviolet light (Wood's light), roughened patches of skin (shagreen patches) usually over the lumbar spine and/or adenoma sebaceum (angiofibromata) in a butterfly distribution over the bridge of the nose and cheeks.

29.10
A. Folic acid ⊘
Correct. Folic acid prior to conception and early in pregnancy significantly reduces the chance of spina bifida (as shown in this image). It is the only vitamin supplement that reduces the risk of neural tube defects.

B. Iron
Iron supplementation is prescribed to treat anaemia during pregnancy.

C. Vitamin A
Vitamin A should not be supplemented in pregnancy as it can harm the developing fetus.

D. Vitamin B_{12}
Vitamin B_{12} is usually only considered if the mother is vegetarian or vegan.

E. Vitamin D
Vitamin D is recommended to be supplemented for healthy bone development.

29.11
A. Childhood Rolandic epilepsy (benign epilepsy with centro-temporal spikes)
This condition comprises 15% of all childhood epilepsies. The EEG shows focal sharp waves from the Rolandic area. Important to recognize as it is relatively benign and may not require antiepileptic drugs. Occurs in 4–10-year-olds and remits in adolescence. Antonia's history does not correspond with this diagnosis. See Table 29.1 in Illustrated Textbook of Paediatrics for more details of epilepsy syndromes.

B. Childhood absence epilepsy ⊘
Correct. The history suggests this diagnosis. In addition, the EEG corresponds with it, showing 3/s spike and wave discharge, which is bilaterally synchronous during, and sometimes between, attacks.

C. Juvenile myoclonic epilepsy
Typically affects 10 to 20 year olds. Antonia's history does not correspond with this diagnosis. See Table 29.1 in Illustrated Textbook of Paediatrics for more details of epilepsy syndromes.

D. Lennox-Gastaut syndrome
This condition affects children 1–3 years old, who have multiple seizure types, but mostly atonic, atypical (subtle) absences and tonic seizures in sleep with neurodevelopmental regression and behaviour disorder. Antonia's history does not correspond with this diagnosis.

E. Infantile spasms (West syndrome)
Antonia's history does not correspond with this diagnosis.

29.12
A. Juvenile myoclonic epilepsy
Vijay's history does not correspond with this diagnosis. See Table 29.1 in Illustrated Textbook of Paediatrics for details of epilepsy syndromes.

B. Lennox-Gastaut syndrome
Vijay's history does not correspond with this diagnosis.

C. Childhood Rolandic epilepsy (benign epilepsy with centro-temporal spikes)
Vijay's history does not correspond with this diagnosis.

D. Childhood absence epilepsy
Wrong age, wrong description and EEG would show three per second spike and wave pattern.

E. Infantile spasms (West syndrome) ⊘
Correct. Vijay has violent flexor spasms of the head, trunk and limbs followed by extension. These are known as infantile spasms. He also has developmental regression. The EEG shown is characteristic, called hypsarrhythmia.

Answers: Extended Matching

Answer 29.13.1
K. Reflex asystolic syncope (reflex anoxic seizure)
These are triggered by pain, often after a trivial fall or knock. The child becomes pale and subsequently may have a generalised tonic–clonic seizure, provoked by hypoxia. This is followed by a rapid recovery and there is no lasting neurological insult. Children with reflex asystolic syncope often have a first-degree relative with a history of faints. A history of breath holding should be sought as it is easy to confuse this with breath-holding attacks.

Answer 29.13.2
L. Syncope
Syncope is often caused by prolonged standing or a prolonged fast. There are often pre-syncopal symptoms, including feeling hot, dizzy and/or visual disturbance. Syncope can lead to jerking movement (clonic movements), which can be mistaken for a seizure.

Answer 29.13.3
C. Cardiac arrhythmia
Warning signs for a cardiac arrhythmia include collapse during exercise, early pallor and a family history of sudden premature death in otherwise fit and healthy relatives. Some types of cardiac arrhythmia (e.g. ventricular tachycardia) have abnormalities present on the ECG e.g long QT, and are provoked by a shock (e.g. diving into a swimming pool). Sometimes there is a structural heart problem (e.g. hypertrophic obstructive cardiomyopathy) that results in ECG changes.

Answer 29.13.4
B. Blue breath-holding spells (expiratory apnoea syncope)
These occur in some upset toddlers. The child will cry, which is immediately followed by an episode of apnoea (breath-holding) and cyanosis, sometimes with loss of consciousness. There is a rapid recovery after such attacks.

Answer 29.13.5
D. Childhood absence epilepsy (typical absence seizure)
Often affected children do not do well at school because of transient loss of consciousness, which impedes learning. They are often described as day-dreamers by their teachers. Absence seizures can be reproduced in the clinical setting by asking the child to hyperventilate for 2 minutes. Asking the child to blow on a toy windmill and keep it spinning quickly or blow out an imaginary candle is helpful (as well as fun).

Answer 29.14.1
A. Childhood Rolandic epilepsy (benign epilepsy with centro-temporal spikes)
This classically presents between the age of 4–10 years, with tonic–clonic seizures in sleep or simple partial seizures, with abnormal feelings in the tongue and distortion of the face. It is also known as benign childhood epilepsy with centro-temporal spikes due to the EEG, which shows focal sharp waves from the Rolandic i.e. centro-temporal area.

Answer 29.14.2
C. Juvenile myoclonic epilepsy
Myoclonic jerks are worse in the morning, especially if the child is sleep deprived. These children may also have generalised tonic–clonic seizures and absences.

Answer 29.14.3
D. Lennox–Gastaut syndrome
Andrew has different seizure types: tonic, atypical absence and atonic seizures. These children often have complex neurological problems and their prognosis is, sadly, very poor. It affects 4% of children with epilepsy and is more common in boys than girls.

Answer 29.15.1
G. Gower's sign
The key to a positive Gower's sign is that the child has to move from a supine to a prone position in order to get up off the floor (this is normal until 3 years of age). It is only later that the classical 'climb up the legs with the hands' feature becomes evident, when muscle weakness is profound. See Fig. 29.6 in Illustrated Textbook of Paediatrics.

Answer 29.15.2
A. Babinski's sign
This comprises upward initial movement of the big toe with or without fanning of the toes. A positive Babinski is normal until 18 months of age. This boy has an upper-motor neurone lesion secondary to perinatal brain injury.

Answer 29.15.3
I. Romberg's sign
The Romberg test is a test of balance. It is performed by asking the child to stand with legs together and arms by the side. The child should then close his/her eyes and be observed for a full minute. Romberg's sign is positive if the patient sways or falls when his/her eyes are closed. Sayeed most likely has Friedreich ataxia. However, this is not a test of cerebellar function, as children with cerebellar ataxia will generally be unable to balance even with their eyes open!

Answer 29.15.4
F. Fogs' sign
Subtle asymmetries in gait may be revealed by Fogs' test – children are asked to walk on their heels, the outside of their feet and then the inside of their feet. Watch for the pattern of abnormal movement in the upper limbs. Observe them running. This girl probably has subtle cerebral palsy, which may be related to her premature birth.

Answer 29.15.5
H. Kernig's sign
Kernig's sign is positive if there is pain on extending the knee. This suggests meningism. To undertake the test, the hip and knee are flexed to 90°. The knee is the extended to 180°. Brudzinski's sign also indicates meningism; the patient should be lying in a supine position and the sign is positive if there is involuntary lifting of the legs when their head is lifted off the couch.

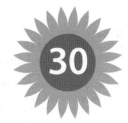

Adolescent medicine

Questions: Single Best Answer

30.1
Which of these Western European countries has the highest incidence of teenage motherhood?

Select one answer only.

A. Denmark
B. France
C. Portugal
D. Spain
E. United Kingdom

30.2
Claire is 15 years old. She visits her general practitioner as she wants to go on the oral contraceptive pill. She is sexually active and has a boyfriend with whom she has been in a relationship for 6 months. Her mother is not aware she has come to see the doctor today, and is also not aware she is sexually active. Claire does not want her mother to know she is getting the oral contraceptive pill. She has no other medical problems. She has regular periods and her blood pressure is normal.

What advice should you give her?

Select one answer only.

A. You will only give her the pill if her parents are present to consent in writing
B. You will prescribe the pill and promise not to tell her parents
C. You will prescribe the pill and encourage her to tell her mother that she is going to start taking the pill
D. You will prescribe the pill but will inform her parents you are doing so
E. She cannot have the pill as she is not legally allowed to have sex

30.3
Which of the following is the most common cause of death in 15–19-year-olds in the UK?

Select one answer only.

A. Malignant disease
B. Heart disease
C. Infection
D. Injury and poisoning
E. Neurological disease

30.4
Olivia is a 16-year-old girl who presents to the local pharmacy for 'emergency contraception'. She has had unprotected sex with her boyfriend, who is also 16 years old. She has no other medical problems and is not currently on any medications.

For how long after unprotected intercourse is emergency contraception effective?

Select one answer only.

A. 12 hours
B. 24 hours
C. 48 hours
D. 72 hours
E. 1 week

Questions: Extended Matching

30.5
From the list of medical disorders encountered in adolescence, select the most likely diagnosis (A–K) for each scenario. Each diagnosis can be used once, more than once, or not at all.

A. Acne vulgaris
B. Asthma
C. Depression
D. Epilepsy
E. Chronic fatigue syndrome
F. Anorexia nervosa
G. Somatic symptoms
H. Risk-taking behaviour (including smoking, drug abuse, alcohol)
I. Pregnancy
J. Malignancy
K. Psychosis

30.5.1

Anika, a 15-year-old girl, presents with her mother to her general practitioner. She complains of vomiting. This is present most often in the morning and is associated with abdominal pain, fatigue, and breast tenderness. You ask her if she has had unprotected sex, and she denies this. She has a suprapubic mass. She has no other medical problems and is not on any medications.

30.5.2

Sam, 16-years-old, is brought to his general practitioner because his parents are worried about him. They complain that he stays locked in his room and is not doing well at school. He often refuses to get out of bed because he has a headache. You speak to Sam alone. He complains of being bored all the time and says that there is nothing he enjoys. He feels hopeless. He no longer goes out with his friends. He complains of a headache, which is of gradual onset and like a tight band around his head. He is a fan of 'ER', a medical drama, is particularly concerned about one of the characters who suffered from a brain tumour. He is convinced that he also has a brain tumour.

30.5.3

Keith, a 15-year-old boy, attends the paediatric outpatient department with his mother. Over the last 6 weeks he has become increasingly aggressive, and last week was suspended from school for throwing his book at a teacher. His mother says that this behaviour is completely out of character; he was previously a kind and hard-working boy. His school performance has also deteriorated. He also complains of an occipital headache that is worse in the morning or when he bends down. His mother sometimes finds vomit in the sink. Examination is normal except for a squint. On checking his eye movements, you find that he is unable to deviate his left eye laterally.

30.5.4

Bennu, a 14-year-old girl whose parents are from Egypt, is sent to the school nurse by her maths teacher because she is complaining of a headache. She complains of a headache at least once a week and often feels tired. There is no pattern to her headaches. She has no other symptoms and is doing well at school. She has lots of friends and is a sociable teenager. There are no abnormalities on examination. She has no other medical problems and is on no medications.

30.5.5

Gareth is a 15-year-old boy who has become increasingly withdrawn. He frequently argues with his mother, particularly when she believes he should stay at home to do his homework rather than leaving the house to meet his new group of friends. His mother believes that this new group of friends are using drugs. She is very upset that he has even been cautioned by the police for urinating in public whilst intoxicated. He has no other medical problems.

Answers: Single Best Answer

30.1

A. Denmark
In 2014 Denmark had the lowest rate of motherhood in the European Union area with rates of 1.1 per 1000 women aged 15–17 years.

B. France
France has a relatively low rate of motherhood with approximately 4.4 births per 1000 young women aged 15–17 in 2014.

C. Portugal
Portugal has reduced rates of motherhood in those under the age of 18 consistently over the last decade and still has rates lower than in the UK. In 2014 these were 5.3 per 1000.

D. Spain
Spain has been consistently one of the better performers in the European Union. Rates remain low but not as low as the Nordic countries and the Netherlands.

E. United Kingdom ⊘
Correct. In 2014 there were 6.8 live births per 1000 young women aged 15–17 in the UK. The highest rates were seen in Bulgaria and Romania with rates of 35.5 per 1000 and 28.2 per 1000 respectively. Data can be found at http://www.ons.gov.uk/ons/dcp171778_353922.pdf for data on conceptions and http://www.ons.gov.uk/ons/rel/vsob1/births-by-area-of-usual-residence-of-mother–england-and-wales/2012/sty-international-comparisons-of-teenage-pregnancy.html for most up to date statistics (Published February 2014).

30.2

C. You will prescribe the pill and encourage her to tell her mother that she is going to start taking the pill ⊘
Correct. It is usually desirable for the parents to be informed and involved in contraception management. She should be encouraged to tell them or allow the doctor to, but if the young person is competent to make these decisions for herself, in the UK the courts have supported medical management of these situations without parental knowledge. This is referred to as Fraser Guidelines (See Chapter 5. Care of the Sick Child and Young Person in Illustrated Textbook of Paediatrics).

30.3

D. Injury and poisoning ⊘
Correct. In the UK, the mortality rate has declined more slowly in adolescents than in other groups. Risk taking behaviour is an important problem, and alcohol is implicated in many cases. Injury and poisoning account for almost half (43%) of deaths in 15–19-year-olds.

30.4

D. 72 hours ⊘
Correct. Emergency contraception is available from a pharmacist without prescription for those aged 16 years and over, and on prescription for those under 16 years. If taken within 72 hours, it has a 2% failure rate.

Answers: Extended Matching

Answer 30.5.1
I. Pregnancy
The symptoms described are of pregnancy. Teenagers often present with symptoms rather than missed periods. She may well deny unprotected sex whilst her mother is present.

Answer 30.5.2
C. Depression
Sam has features of depression including apathy, inability to enjoy himself, decline in school performance and hypochondriacal ideas. His headache is most likely a tension headache.

Answer 30.5.3
J. Malignancy
Keith has symptoms of a brain tumour. His behaviour has changed, and he has a headache suggestive of raised intracranial pressure. The squint is a VI nerve palsy, a 'false-localizing sign' of raised intracranial pressure. Fundoscopy and blood pressure measurement should be undertaken and he should have an urgent brain scan.

Answer 30.5.4
G. Somatic symptoms
Bennu has no symptoms of depression, and there are no associated danger signs ('red-flag' signs) with the headache. Somatic symptoms are common in teenagers, with 25% complaining of headache more than once a week.

Answer 30.5.5
H. Risk-taking behaviour
Gareth has started to explore 'adult' behaviours including smoking, drinking and drug use. These 'risk-taking' behaviours reflect Gareth's search for new and enjoyable experiences, as well as exerting independence from his mother and rebelling against her wishes.

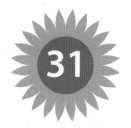

Global child health

Questions: Single Best Answer

31.1
Worldwide, which of the following conditions is most likely to result in the death of an individual child before their fifth birthday?

Select one answer only.

A. Gastroenteritis
B. HIV (Human immunodeficiency virus) infection
C. Injuries
D. Malaria
E. Prematurity

31.2
Worldwide, which of the following factors is most important in predicting neonatal mortality?

Select one answer only.

A. Birth order
B. Household wealth
C. Maternal educational achievement
D. Paternal educational achievement
E. Urban versus rural residency

31.3
Which of the following causes of death in childhood is likely to increase most in the next 15 years?

Select one answer only.

A. HIV infection
B. Malaria
C. Malnutrition
D. Pneumonia
E. Trauma

Answers: Single Best Answer

31.1

A. Gastroenteritis
This is a very important cause of morbidity but since the 1970s and the widespread use of oral rehydration solution, deaths from gastroenteritis have fallen. It is now responsible for 9% of deaths of children under 5 years of age.

B. HIV infection
A worldwide catastrophe that shows signs of improvement. Prevention of mother to child transmission has helped considerably. It is now responsible for 1% of deaths of children under 5 years of age.

C. Injuries
This is the leading cause of death in older children. Globally, it is responsible for 6% of deaths of children under 5 years of age.

D. Malaria
An important treatable cause of death. It is now responsible for 5% of deaths of children under 5 years of age.

E. **Prematurity** ⊘
Correct. Prematurity accounts for 16% of deaths in children under 5 years of age. Overall, 44% of all deaths occur in the neonatal period and of these prematurity is the leading cause. Pneumonia is the next most common cause of death, responsible for 13% of all deaths in children under 5.

31.2

A. Birth order
Birth order does affect childhood mortality but the effect is small.

B. Household wealth
There is still a difference in neonatal mortality according to wealth but it is less than the differences from maternal educational achievement.

C. **Maternal educational achievement** ⊘
Correct. A well-educated mother is much less likely to have a neonatal death than a poorly educated one. See Figure 31.3 in Illustrated Textbook of Paediatrics for comparisons between different 'modifiable' factors.

D. Paternal educational achievement
This has an effect but is not as marked as the effect of maternal education.

E. Urban versus rural residency
Urban living is associated with lower mortality but the effect is less than that seen in maternal education.

31.3

A. HIV infection
Death in children from HIV infection should not increase because of prevention of mother to child transmission and increasing availability and efficacy of treatment.

B. Malaria
Mortality from malaria is decreasing because of insecticide-treated bed nets, mosquito control, and early treatment, often by community health workers.

C. Malnutrition
Food poverty is an important problem but it is not predicted to increase.

D. Pneumonia
Pneumonia is a major cause of death during childhood. It is particularly important in younger children but is not increasing.

E. **Trauma** ⊘
Correct. Mortality from unintentional injury, mainly through road traffic incidents, is predicted to increase.

Index

Page numbers followed by "*f*" indicate figures, "*t*" indicate tables, and "*b*" indicate boxes.

A

Abdomen
 ultrasound of, 34, 38, 126, 130
 X-ray of, 35, 38
ABO incompatibility, 65, 68
Accidental injury, 40, 40f, 43
Accidents
 burns, 34, 35f, 38
 poisoning and, 33-39
Achondroplasia, autosomal dominant disorder, 48-49, 54
Acute lymphoblastic leukaemia, 7
Adolescent medicine, 177
Adrenal tumour, 70, 72
Advice, for emotional and behavioural problems, 139, 141
Airway opening manoeuvres, paediatric emergencies and, 28, 32
Alcohol, 36, 39
Allergy, 93-94
 Cow's milk protein, 11
Analgesia, 88-89, 92
 intravenous, 34, 38
Anaphylaxis, 93-94
Anorexia nervosa, 138, 140
Anti-epileptic drug therapy, 168-169, 174
Antibiotics, for leukaemia, 124, 128
Antipyretic, 88-89, 92
Aorta, coarctation of, 106, 108
Aortic stenosis, 105-106, 105f, 108-109
Apgar score, 57, 61
Appendicitis, 80, 84
Arthritis
 reactive, 160, 162, 165-166
 septic, 159-160, 162, 164, 166
 systemic-onset juvenile idiopathic, 160, 165
ASD. *see* Atrial septal defect (ASD)
Asthma, 1-2, 96, 101
 history and examination of, 6, 6f, 8
Ataxic (hypotonic) cerebral palsy, developmental problems and, 16, 20
Atopic eczema, 146, 146f, 149
Atresia, biliary, 121, 123
Atrial septal defect (ASD), 105-106, 105f, 108
Atrioventricular septal defect, 46, 50
Auditory brainstem response audiometry, 11
Autism spectrum disorder
 age of, 13, 18
 developmental problems and, 13, 18
Autoimmune pancreatic β-cell damage, 150, 154
Autonomy, for child, 23, 25

Autosomal dominant disorder
 achondroplasia, 48-49, 54
 Marfan syndrome, 49, 54, 54t
Autosomal dominant inheritance, 47, 47f, 52
Autosomal recessive disorder, sickle cell disease, 49, 54
Autosomal recessive inheritance, 46, 46f, 51

B

Babinski sign, 172, 176
Baby, assessment of, 152-153, 152f, 156
Bacterial infection, in eczema, 143, 148
Bacterial meningitis, 85, 90
Balanoposthitis, broad-spectrum antibiotic and warm baths for, 117, 119
Barrel chest, 7-8
Basal ganglia lesion, 7
Beneficence, sick child and, 23, 25
Benign epilepsy, with centro-temporal spikes. *see* Childhood Rolandic epilepsy
Benzoyl peroxide, topical, for acne, 143, 143f, 148
Biliary atresia, 65, 68, 121, 123
Bilirubin, level of, 63, 67
Biopsy, excision, 127, 130
Birth order, neonatal mortality and, 180-181
Birthweight, cardiovascular disease and, 74, 76
Bite marks, non-accidental injury and, 41, 41f, 44
Blood culture, for leukaemia, 124, 128
Blood glucose
 hepatomegaly and, 120, 122
 for hypoglycaemia, 29, 32
 level, paediatric emergencies and, 28, 31
 measurements of, 150, 151f, 154
Blood tests, for assessment of baby, 152-153, 152f, 156
Blood transfusion, 133, 136
Blue breath-holding spells (expiratory apnoea syncope), 171, 176
Bone fracture, parietal, 33, 33f, 37, 37f
Bone marrow aspirate, 126, 130
Bordetella pertussis, 95, 100
Bow legs-rickets, 163, 167
BPD. *see* Bronchopulmonary dysplasia (BPD)
Brain, CT or MRI scan of, 15, 19
Brain tumour, 126, 130
Breast milk
 disadvantages of, 74-75, 77
 jaundice, 65, 68
Broad-spectrum antibiotic, for balanoposthitis, 117, 119
Bronchiolitis, 98, 102
 history and examination of, 5, 5f, 8
Bronchopulmonary dysplasia (BPD), 65, 65f, 68, 98, 98f, 102
Buccal glucose gel, 150, 154
Burns, 34, 35f, 38
 'glove and stocking' distribution of, 42, 42f, 44